THE ART of LONGEVITY:
MY TRUE-LIFE STORY, HEALTH - SPAN and SCIENCE

Sterling Blessworth

CHAPTER I

INTRODUCTION

I am 70 years now with two children. When I was 30 years old – pregnant with my second child, I was discovering that I have the Diabetes disease from my father. My father passed away when he was 30 years old. Due to my father, I was more likely to develop the diabetes disease. So, there will be more likely my two children to develop diabetes as well and so on, including to my future grandchildren.

"Then to be told that this might be the thing that might take you out was like, its kind a floored me", that was my thought back then.

Due to life-altering diagnosis of Type 2 diabetes for myself and a chance to my children and my future grandchildren, I have studied a lot about this disease.

across to all science, lifestyle, habit & Ikigai, diet & nutrition – Blue Zones, exercise, sleep management, emotional health and more. One of my sons has been working in a company in California USA with 700+ Providers & Facilities in Network. This company to transform healthcare by focusing on "well care" rather than traditional "sick care." By embracing Lifestyle Medicine principles, they treat the whole person—addressing diet, exercise, sleep, and stress—before resorting to medications and surgery. Their goal is **to create a happier, healthier you.**

This is how I see my role: telling you my true life story with help of my son, helping you understand and apply this insight to empower you to reverse your disease with "well care," before resorting to medications and/or surgery. **And you may get "BIG BONUS" with LONGEVITY AND HEALTHSPAN as well.** Lifespan is the number of years someone lives from birth until death, while health span is the number of years someone is healthy without chronic and debilitating disease.

I do hope that you will learn and get the benefit of my extraordinary journey by reading this book. My odyssey takes an unexpected turn when, just a few years into my diabetes diagnosis, I stumbled upon a remote village nestled deep in the heart of a Mediterranean island. What I discovered there not only reshapes my perspective on longevity but also leaves an indelible mark on my own quest for health span. In this remote village, I encountered a community of centenarians, individuals living well into their hundreds, with a vigor and vitality that defy the passage of time.

What is their secret?

I delved into their daily lives, a symphony of habits, diets, and philosophies that have been honed over centuries. The first revelation is their diet. These centenarians consume a rich Mediterranean diet, replete with colorful vegetables, heart-healthy olive oil, and lean protein sources like fish and legumes. Their plates are a canvas of nature's bounty, and the science behind this diet is compelling. Research consistently demonstrates the Mediterranean diet's ability to reduce the risk of chronic diseases and promote longevity. But diet is only one piece of the puzzle. My journey takes me deeper into the fabric of their existence, revealing their daily rituals of physical activity. These centenarians are not marathon runners; instead, they engage in gentle, purposeful movement—whether it is tending to their gardens or taking leisurely walks along the coastal cliffs. The science here is irrefutable: regular, low- impact physical activity contributes significantly to health span, reducing the risk of chronic diseases and improving overall well-being.

However, it is the philosophy of these centenarians that strikes the most profound chord. They embrace a life lived slowly and intentionally, cherishing the moments, cultivating deep social connections, and nurturing a powerful sense of purpose (Ikigai in Japanese culture).

The science supports this, too: positive social interactions, a sense of belonging, and a clear sense of purpose are critical factors in promoting a long and fulfilling life. As you immerse yourself in this book, my story encountered with these remarkable centenarians becomes a rallying cry, urging you to take charge of your own health span journey. You will find yourself inspired to adopt the principles of their Mediterranean lifestyle, weaving vibrant, nutrient-rich foods into your diet, incorporating gentle movement into your daily routine, and nurturing a sense of purpose and social connection.

I also came to Japan to do some research in Okinawa, where Okinawa is one of The BLUE ZONES. They have some similarity LIFESTYLE as in Mediterranean island as discussed earlier. Such as their diet, IKIGAI, gentle exercise by walking. As we know, most Japanese use

Public Transport most days due to their system and infrastructure. They must do a lot of steps daily from their home to station and to their office also back home of course. For them, this is a kind of DEFAULT, they must do this, but this condition has a great benefit for them.

Japanese's diet also having interesting character, which are **A LOT OF FRESH**: they get the food material still fresh (vegetables, meat, fish, even noddle all in FRESH condition), cook and eat while still FRESH as well. It is hardly to find a process food over there. Not to mention, they are eating a lot of fish.

With each chapter in this book, you will find that my narrative becomes a roadmap, guiding you towards a life marked by not just longevity, but health span—a life filled with energy, vitality, and the wisdom to savor each moment. This book is more than a memoir; it is a call to action, a scientific exploration, and an invitation to embark on your own journey towards a vibrant, resilient, and fulfilling life.

We have several friend, man, and women in their 50s and 60s. They are gaining weight, easy to get exhausted, have some medical condition, not a happy person and have some aches as well. These friends are easier to get sick and take much longer than usual to recover than other people. These friends believe that their condition is unavoidable and they think it is a given of The Normal Aging of human being.

On the other hand, we have a bunch of other friends who we thought was forties and turned out to be 60s. Most people thought that I was fifties, but actually I am 70 years because I am practicing **all the TIPS OF HABITS, DIET, EXERCISE, SLEEPING, LIFESTYLE AND MORE** which are discussed in this book.

So, we have TWO GROUP here, Group Healthy is a group of people who aged amazingly well, looking great, feeling well, happy, strong, healthy, and energetic.

In this book we help you to become one of The Group Healthy as well. This book guides you to reversing disease, easing pain, and living younger longer.

Aging has been considered as a normal process. We think frailty and gradual decline are inevitable parts of life. They do not have to be. Science sees aging as a treatable disease. We do need to address to its root causes, and we will increase our health span, live longer, and reverse the illness of aging. Aging is not just about living long. It is **ALSO** about being happy, to be able still doing things we love, looking and feeling well.

You are becoming Your Own Personal Wellness Coach for yourself. How you age, in many ways, is **UP TO YOU.** The good news, it is never too late to start with A NEW HABITS, NEW DIET and LIFESTYLE to get A GREAT IMPROVEMENT OF YOUR HEALTH JOURNEY.

In this book, we uncover the secrets to longevity, we explore the biological of aging, their causes, and their consequences. We also show you how to overcome them with dietary, lifestyle, exercises, longevity strategies and much more. So, you can turn on your key longevity switches with several activities including The Blue Zones Diet, Ikigai and about eating 80 % FULL **(Hara Hachi Bu)** as well.

Aging is a complex and multi-factorial process that affects every living organism. As we age, our bodies undergo a variety of changes that can impact our overall health and well-being. While aging is maybe inevitable, but the rate at which we age and the degree to which we experience age-related health issues can vary greatly.

Recent research has shown that aging is not simply a result of the passage of time, but rather a complex interplay between genetics, lifestyle, environmental factors and more. Studies have revealed that a significant percentage of the aging process is under epigenetic control, meaning that lifestyle and environmental factors can modify our gene expression, leading to aging-related diseases.

The good news is that by understanding the science of aging, we can take steps to promote healthy aging and maximize our longevity. An integrated approach to aging, which recognizes that all aspects of our lives – including nutrition, exercise, stress management, sleep, and social support – are interconnected and play a role in aging, is the key to achieving healthy aging. By taking an integrated approach to aging, we can address all these factors and create a comprehensive plan for maximizing our longevity and well-being.

Nutrition plays a critical role in aging, as the foods we eat can impact our overall health and well-being in a number of ways. Eating a diet that is rich in whole foods, such as fruits, vegetables, lean protein, and healthy fats, can help to support healthy aging by providing the body with the essential nutrients it needs to function at its best. Adequate intake of antioxidants, vitamins, and minerals are also important to combat the effects of free radicals and inflammation which are associated with aging. Furthermore, the role of nutraceuticals such as resveratrol and curcumin, which have been shown to have anti-aging properties, are areas of ongoing research.

Exercise is also a vital component of healthy aging, as regular physical activity can help to improve cardiovascular health, increase muscle mass and strength, and boost overall energy levels. Regular exercise can also help to improve the health of our bones, boost our immune system, and reduce the risk of chronic diseases such as diabetes and heart disease. Additionally, exercise has been shown to promote the activation of anti-aging pathways such as the sirtuins and improve the function of mitochondria, the powerhouses of our cells.

Stress management is another important aspect of healthy aging, as elevated levels of stress can take a toll on both our physical and mental health. Chronic stress has been linked to a variety of health problems including high blood pressure, heart disease, and depression. By learning how to manage stress and cultivate a sense of calm and well-being, we can help to promote healthy aging. Mindfulness practices such as meditation and yoga can be effective tools in managing stress. Additionally, understanding the impact of chronic stress on our hormone balance, particularly cortisol and its impact on inflammation, is critical in the management of stress.

Sleep is also critical for healthy aging, as it allows our bodies to repair and rejuvenate. Adequate sleep is essential for maintaining a healthy immune system, cognitive function, and overall physical well-being. By getting enough quality sleep each night, we can help to support healthy aging and improve our overall well-being. Additionally, studies have shown that certain sleep patterns, such as the presence of deep sleep, are associated with healthier aging.

Also Social Support can also play a role in aging, as having a strong network of friends and loved ones can help to promote a sense of well-being and improve overall health. Studies have shown that people with strong social support networks is aging beautifully.

This book is about a comprehensive guide to understanding the numerous factors that contribute to the aging process and how a comprehensive approach to healthy living can promote longevity. This book delves into the latest research and findings in the field of aging, providing detailed information on the various biological, psychological, and environmental factors that affect aging.

One of the key concepts discussed in the book is the idea of **Ikigai,** which is a Japanese term that refers to one's sense of purpose or meaning in life. Having a powerful sense of Ikigai can lead to a happier and more fulfilling life, which in turn can promote better health and longevity. To support this argument, in Chapter II, you can read a case study of individuals who have found their Ikigai and have seen significant improvements in their health and well-being as a result.

Another important topic covered in the book is the diet and lifestyle habits of people living in **"blue zones,"** which are areas around the world where people have been found to live longer and healthier lives. This book provides detailed information on the specific dietary and lifestyle practices of these populations and how they contribute to longevity. For example, you can read the traditional diet of the Okinawan people of Japan, which is characterized by a high consumption of sweet potatoes, tofu, and green leafy vegetables, and is associated with lower rates of chronic diseases and longevity.

This book also covers other crucial factors such as genetics, stress management, and environment and how they all interplay to impact health and lifespan.

The author provides strategies and tips on how to manage stress, a case study of the impact of environment on human health and longevity. As you may know a story of a man who moved from a polluted city to a small town and as a result, he has seen a significant improvement in his lung function and overall health.

Overall, this book is a comprehensive and informative guide to understanding the science of aging and the many ways in which a comprehensive approach to health and well-being can promote longevity. It provides detailed information on the latest research and findings in the field and uses case studies and real-life examples to illustrate the importance of a comprehensive approach to aging and longevity. Whether you are a healthcare professional, a researcher, or simply someone who is interested in living a longer, healthier life, this book is a valuable resource that will provide you with the knowledge and tools you need to take a more comprehensive approach to aging and longevity.

With a lot of science-based strategies and tips, this Book is a revolutionary, practical guide to creating and sustaining health—for life.
To get THE GREAT BENEFIT OF THIS BOOK to address to its root causes, so you will increase your health

span, live longer, and reverse the illness of aging, please read all chapters from Chapter I until Chapter XVIII. Remember Aging is not just about living long. It is **ALSO** about being happy, to be able still doing things we love, looking and feeling well (HEALTH-SPAN).

<u>WHY NOT WE GET THIS TOGETHER?</u>

CHAPTER II

THE ROLE OF MINDFULNESS IN ANTI-AGING, INCLUDING IKIGAI

Mindfulness have been shown to have numerous benefits for overall health and well-being, and recent research suggests that they may also play a role in anti-aging.

One of the main ways that mindfulness can help to promote anti-aging is by reducing stress and inflammation. Chronic stress can lead to an increase in inflammation throughout the body, which can contribute to the development of chronic diseases such as heart disease, diabetes, and cancer. Mindfulness have been shown to reduce stress by decreasing the activity of the stress hormone cortisol and promoting relaxation.

Mindfulness also have been shown to improve cardiovascular health. A study published in JAMA Internal Medicine found that a mindfulness-based stress reduction program led to a significant reduction in blood pressure and improved heart rate variability in participants with hypertension. Another study published in the journal Circulation found that mindfulness may reduce the risk of heart disease by reducing inflammation and improving the function of blood vessels.

Mindfulness also can improve cognitive function, which is important for maintaining a healthy brain and preventing age-related cognitive decline. A study published in Frontiers in Aging Neuroscience found that mindfulness may improve cognitive function, including attention and working memory, in older adults.

In addition, mindfulness has been shown to improve overall well-being and quality of life, which can help to promote healthy aging. A study published in JAMA Internal Medicine found that a mindfulness-based stress reduction program led to improved mood and quality of life in participants with chronic health conditions.

There have been many scientific studies conducted in recent years on the relationship between mindfulness and anti-aging. One of the most recent studies is a randomized controlled trial published in the journal JAMA Network Open in 2019. The study included 98 adults aged 55 to 85 who were randomly assigned to either a mindfulness-based stress reduction (MBSR) program or a health education control group. The MBSR program included eight weekly sessions of mindfulness practices such as body scan and yoga, as well as a one-day retreat.

The study found that the MBSR group had significantly lower levels of the biomarkers of cellular aging, known as telomeres, compared to the control group. Telomeres are the protective caps on the ends of chromosomes that shorten as we age, and shorter telomeres have been linked with a higher risk of age-related diseases and early death. The study also found that the MBSR group had significantly lower levels of inflammation, compared to the control group.

Another recent study published in the journal Aging and Mental Health in 2019, included sixty adults aged sixty and older who were randomly assigned to either a mindfulness-based stress reduction program or a waitlist control group. The study found that the MBSR group had significantly lower levels of inflammation, compared to the control group. The study also found that the MBSR group had improved cognitive function, including working memory, attention, and executive function, compared to the control group.

In conclusion, these recent studies provide convincing evidence that mindfulness and meditation can have anti-aging benefits by reducing stress, inflammation.

IKIGAI

Ikigai is a Japanese concept that refers to the reason for being, the thing that gets you out of bed in the morning and gives you a sense of purpose and fulfilment. The word "ikigai" is made up of two Japanese characters: "iki" meaning "life" and "gai" meaning "value" or "worth." In other words, ikigai is the value or worth of your life. Ikigai is often represented by a Venn diagram with four overlapping circles: what

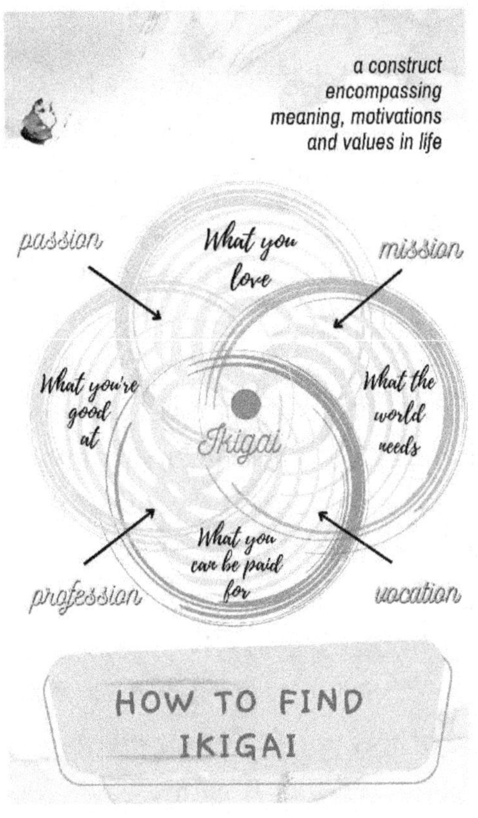

you love, what you are good at, what the world needs, and for what you can be paid. Finding your ikigai is considered essential for living a fulfilling life and for achieving a sense of balance and happiness.

The idea of ikigai is rooted in the Japanese culture and philosophy that emphasizes the importance of living a purposeful and meaningful life. It is a way of finding your own unique path and making the most of your talents and passions.

One of the key principles of ikigai is the idea of "flow," which is a state of mind in which you are completely absorbed in an activity and lose track of time. According to the concept of ikigai, flow can be achieved when you are doing something that you love, that you are good at, and that is meaningful to you.

Ikigai also emphasizes the importance of living in harmony with others and with the environment. It encourages people to be mindful and present in their daily lives, and to seek connection and community. Some people find their ikigai through their work, others through their hobbies, and still others through their relationships or community service. The key is to find something that brings you joy and fulfilment and that aligns with your values and passions.

There is some evidence to suggest that having a sense of purpose and fulfilment in life, as embodied by the concept of ikigai, may contribute to better health and potentially even longevity.

Studies have shown that people who have a sense of purpose in life tend to have better physical and mental health and are less likely to develop chronic conditions such as heart disease, diabetes, and depression. They also tend to have stronger immune systems and better cognitive function.

Additionally, having a sense of purpose and fulfilment in life can also help to reduce stress and inflammation, which are both factors that can contribute to aging. Stress is known to accelerate the aging process, and chronic inflammation is associated with a wide range of age-related diseases.

Moreover, having a sense of purpose and fulfilment in life can also help to improve overall well-being, which can help to promote healthy aging. People who have a sense of purpose and fulfilment in life tend to have better mood and quality of life and are more likely to be engaged in their communities and to have strong social connections. Social connections are one of the most important predictors of health and longevity, as people with strong social connections tend to live longer and have better physical and mental health.

In conclusion, having a sense of purpose and fulfilment in life, as embodied by the concept of ikigai, may contribute to better health and potentially even longevity.

There is an example of a Japanese man who practices ikigai in his daily life. His name is Mr. Tanaka, a retired businessperson who lives in Utsunomiya, a small town in Japan. After working for many years in the corporate world, Mr. Tanaka decided to retire early to pursue his passion for gardening. He has always loved working with plants and has a particular interest in traditional Japanese gardening techniques.

When he retired, he decided to start a small garden design business, focusing on creating traditional Japanese gardens for his clients. He loved the idea of being able to use his skills and knowledge to create beautiful gardens that bring joy to others, and it was a way to share his passion with the world.

He starts his day early, waking up at 5 a.m. to do a short meditation session, which helps him to clear his mind and focus for the day ahead. He then spends the morning working in his own garden, tending to the plants, pruning, and making sure everything is in order. After lunch, he visits his clients, discussing their garden plans and making suggestions on how to enhance the beauty and serenity of their gardens. He finds great satisfaction in creating beautiful gardens that not only bring joy to his clients but also create a sense of harmony and balance in their lives. In the evening, he takes a walk around his neighbourhood, admiring the different gardens and taking inspiration for his own work. He finds that the simple act of walking and being in nature helps him to clear his mind and feel more connected to the world around him.

Mr. Tanaka's ikigai lies at the intersection of his passion for gardening, his skills and knowledge in traditional Japanese gardening techniques, the needs of his clients, and the fact that he can be paid for it. He found something that makes him happy, he is good at it as well.

Mr. Tanaka is in his early seventies. He has been practicing ikigai for several years now and he has noticed that since he started his garden design business and incorporating ikigai into his daily life, he feels more fulfilled and happier, and his overall well-being has improved. He has a good relationship with his clients, and always receive positive feedback from them. Moreover, he has been more active and has more energy than before. He always says that ikigai has helped him to age gracefully and find joy in his daily life.

CHAPTER III

THE POWER OF NUTRITION: EATING FOR A LONG AND HEALTHY LIFE

This chapter delves into the latest research and findings on the impact of nutrition on aging, providing detailed information on the specific dietary practices and nutrient intake that can promote longevity.

our gut microbiome is the home of trillions of bacteria and other microbes that live in your gut. These microbes influence your digestion, immune system, and skin health. Now when you consume junk food, which is high in sugar and fat, you may strain your microbiome, resulting in poor digestion, immunity, skin quality and so on. Along with junk food, alcohol consumption can have a similar impact.

On the other hand, eating probiotic foods could boost your gut health. The expert recommended consuming foods packed with beneficial bacteria, such as kombucha, live yogurt, tempeh, kimchi and kefir. The expert added that foods packed with antioxidant compounds, such as cacao, pomegranates, berries, almonds, and spinach, could also benefit your microbiome and overall longevity.

A balanced diet is especially important for overall health and wellness. The diet that is rich in fruits, vegetables, whole grains, and lean proteins is essential for maintaining a healthy weight, reducing the risk of chronic diseases, and promoting healthy aging. It is scientific research that shows how reducing calorie intake may slow down aging and increase lifespan.

It is importance of consuming adequate amounts of antioxidants, such as vitamins C and E, for protecting against cellular damage and inflammation, which are both associated with aging. Also it is importance of consuming enough omega-3 fatty acids for maintaining cognitive function and reducing the risk of dementia.

There are several types of diet, such as The Mediterranean diet, which is characterized by a high consumption of fruits, vegetables, whole grains, and fish, and is associated with lower rates of chronic diseases and longer life expectancy. Another one which is more popular is The Blue zones diet, which is a term that refers to the dietary patterns of people who live in the so-called "blue zones" around the world **where people tend to live longer and healthier lives.**

The blue zones are areas in the world: Loma Linda – California USA, Sardinia – Italy, Ikaria – Greece, Okinawa – Japan, and Nicoya – Costa Rica. These areas are far from each other, but they all have a few things in common regarding the people's longevity of life and health. They follow some simple culinary rules, and this has widely become known as the blue zone diet. The guideline is mainly to eat fresh, not processed.

Whole foods only, this should be a number one goal when eating food on the blue zone diet, not the processed stuff. See the details as below:

BEANS

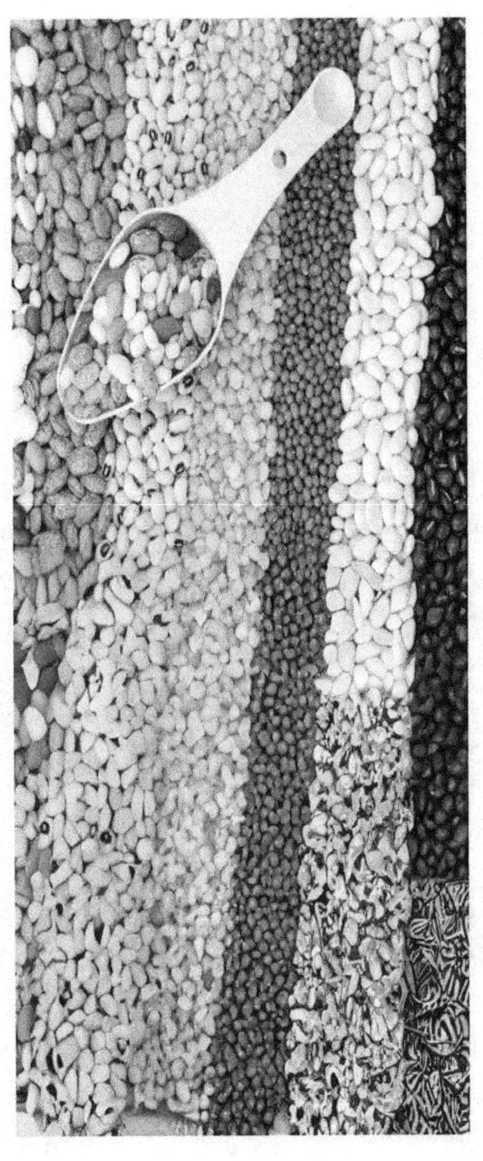

Beans are so good for you. For the blue zone way of eating one cup of beans can be mixed with your meals throughout the day, in a salad, in a stew or curry, on toast or any other food. Tofu is also in this category, as well as beans they contain an excellent quality amount of Fiber and protein.

FISH

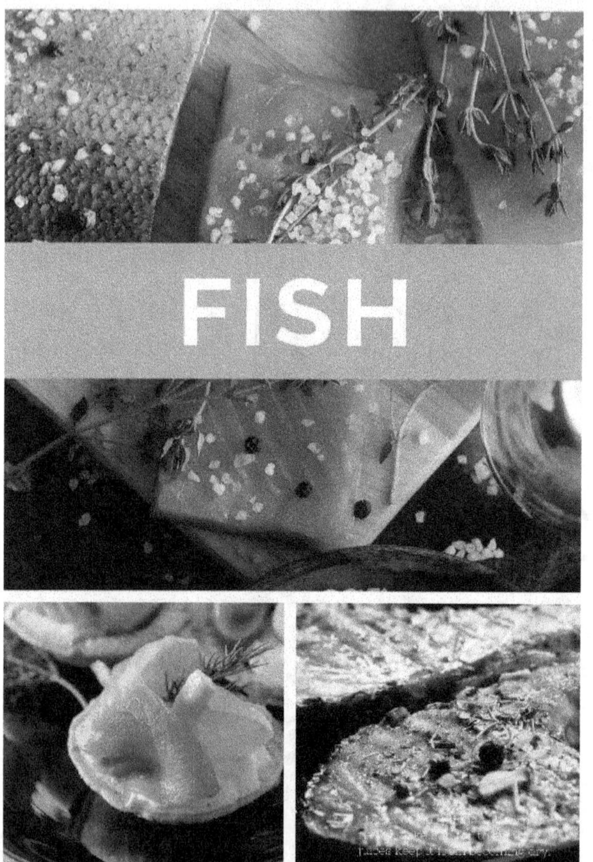

They encourage you to eating fish, up to three times per week. Fish is a wonderful and nutrition white meat, it is low in saturated fats and some fish have health benefits. Choose fish such as wild caught salmon (NOT farmed salmon). Another fish are cod, snapper, trout, sardines, and anchovies. These have good Omega 3 fatty acids, it is beneficial to the function of the human body. The Portion size for fish is around three ounces.

VEGETABLES

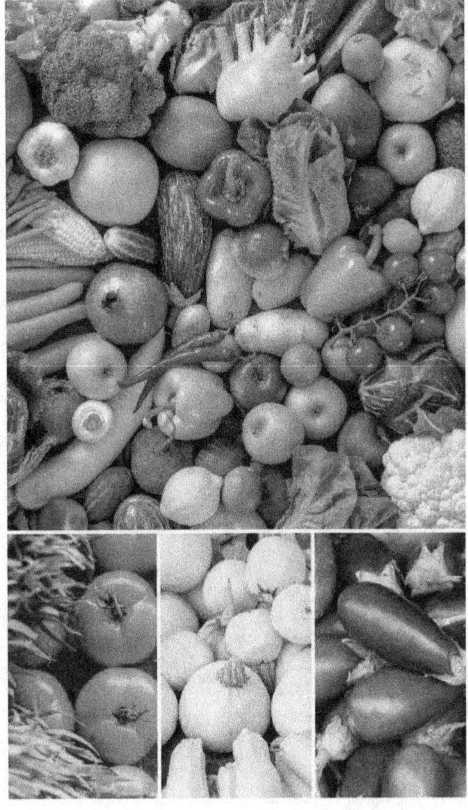

Plants and vegetables are so good for the human body. Apparently these plants and vegetable has protein. Plant foods even have a better, more concentrated, protein element than that which is found in animal foods. On the other hand animal protein contains extra stuff like cholesterol, saturated fats, and even antibiotics and added hormones. Consuming all kinds of fruits and vegetables is one of the first tips for this way of eating, but getting down to specifics, green leafy vegetables are the best regarding nutrition. For fruit, on the Blue Zones Diet, there is no limit on which fruits you can eat.

MEAT

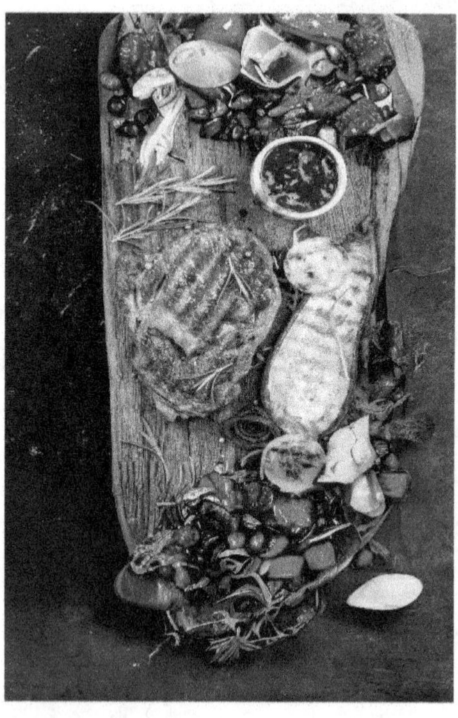

The Blue zone diet does not cut out meat entirely. For those who still enjoy beef, chicken or pork, a wonderful way to incorporate them into this way of eating is to limit your consumption of meat to eat it only once, twice per week. Think of them as a CEREMONIAL FOOD! Remember we are talking quality cuts of meat here, no processed meat food!

DAIRY

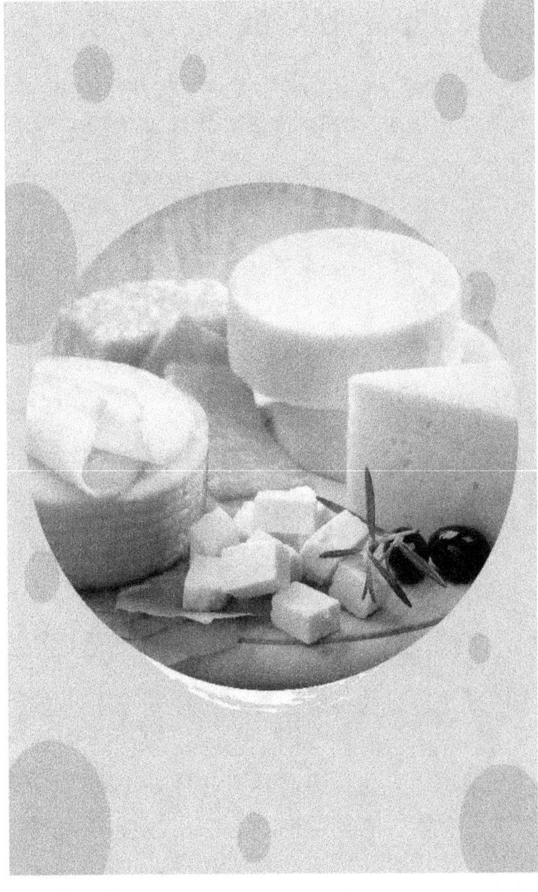

It is not encouraged for eating on this blue zone eating plan, please avoid it if you can. If you cannot, reduce it. Take a goat feta or pecorino, as they are full of flavour and lower in calories and fat, than cheese from cow's milk. A great alternative is coconut milk or almond milk. Eggs can be limited to three times a week.

SUGAR

You may do not realize that sugar is in many products, so please read the labels. Ideally, you should slash your sugar intake as less as possible. You can use honey as a sweetener in many things that you would normally add sugar to. If possible cut out the cookies, cakes, and candies.

BREAD

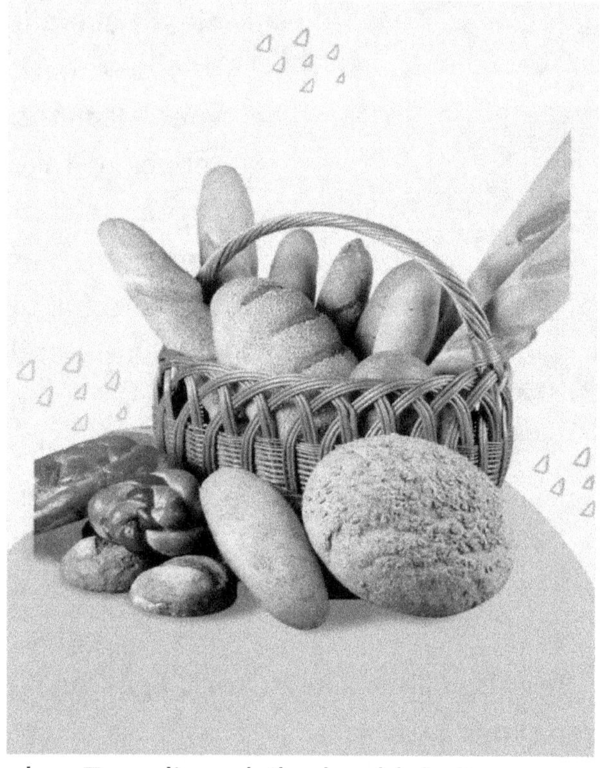

Stick to 100% whole grain bread and avoid the white bread and white flour tortillas. Sourdough bread is also good on this blue zone eating plan. Two slices daily should do it.

NUTS

Best to eat a mix of nuts a couple of handfuls per day,

such as Almonds, walnuts, pistachios, sunflower seeds or pumpkin seeds, brazil nuts, cashews, peanuts. Eating in moderation and mixing up your choice of nuts is the key to not getting bored. Do not forget to eat unsalted nut and not to eat the sugar-coated nuts.

THE OKINAWAN DIET (ONE OF THE BLUE ZONES)

It is a traditional dietary pattern that is characterized by a high consumption of sweet potatoes, tofu, and green leafy vegetables, and is associated with lower rates of chronic diseases and longevity. The diet is also low in animal protein, and it emphasizes on the consumption of plant-based foods. Here is a sample of a 7-day meal plan for the Okinawan diet that includes breakfast, lunch, and dinner:

Day 1:
- Breakfast: Sweet potato and vegetable stir-fry with tofu
- Lunch: Brown rice with mixed vegetables, seaweed and tofu
- Dinner: Grilled fish with a side of mixed vegetables and brown rice

Day 2:
- Breakfast: Sweet potato and vegetable frittata with a side of mixed greens

- Lunch: Brown rice with mixed vegetables, seaweed and tofu
- Dinner: Vegetable and tofu curry with brown rice

Day 3:

- Breakfast: Sweet potato and vegetable hash with a side of poached eggs
- Lunch: Brown rice with mixed vegetables, seaweed and tofu
- Dinner: Baked fish with a side of mixed vegetables and brown rice

Day 4:

- Breakfast: Sweet potato and vegetable smoothie bowl with a sprinkle of sesame seeds
- Lunch: Brown rice with mixed vegetables, seaweed and tofu
- Dinner: Stir-fry of vegetables with tofu and brown rice

Day 5:

- Breakfast: Sweet potato and vegetable omelette with a side of mixed greens
- Lunch: Brown rice with mixed vegetables, seaweed and tofu
- Dinner: Grilled fish with a side of mixed vegetables and brown rice

Day 6:

- Breakfast: Sweet potato and vegetable pancakes with a side of mixed nuts
- Lunch: Brown rice with mixed vegetables, seaweed and tofu
- Dinner: Stir-fry of vegetables with tofu and brown rice

Day 7:

- Breakfast: Sweet potato and vegetable porridge with a sprinkle of sesame seeds
- Lunch: Brown rice with mixed vegetables, seaweed and tofu
- Dinner: Grilled fish with a side of mixed vegetables and brown rice

It is worth noting that this is just an example of what a 7-day Okinawan diet meal plan might look like. You can adjust based on personal preferences and dietary restrictions, if you stick to the general principles of the Okinawan Diet.

The other dietary patterns and their relationship with longevity is The DASH diet.

THE DASH (Dietary Approaches to Stop Hypertension) DIET

It is an eating pattern that is designed to lower blood pressure and reduce the risk of cardiovascular disease. The diet is rich in fruits, vegetables, whole grains, lean proteins, and low-fat dairy products, and it is also low in saturated fat, cholesterol, and added sugars. Here is a sample of a 7-day meal plan for the DASH diet that includes breakfast, lunch, and dinner.

Day 1:
- Breakfast: Oatmeal with banana slices and almond milk
- Lunch: Grilled chicken breast with mixed greens salad and a balsamic vinaigrette
- Dinner: Baked salmon with roasted vegetables and quinoa

Day 2:
- Breakfast: Greek yogurt with berries and a sprinkle of flaxseed
- Lunch: Turkey and avocado wrap with mixed greens and tomato
- Dinner: Whole wheat spaghetti with marinara sauce and turkey meatballs

Day 3:
- Breakfast: Scrambled eggs with spinach and tomato, whole wheat toast

- Lunch: Black bean and corn salad, mixed greens with balsamic vinaigrette
- Dinner: Grilled chicken breast with a side of roasted sweet potatoes

Day 4:
- Breakfast: Whole wheat English muffin with peanut butter and banana slices
- Lunch: Grilled chicken breast with a side of mixed greens salad and balsamic vinaigrette
- Dinner: Stir-fry of vegetables with tofu and brown rice

Day 5:
- Breakfast: Whole wheat toast with avocado and egg
- Lunch: Turkey and cheese sandwich on whole wheat bread with mixed greens and tomato
- Dinner: Baked chicken breast with a side of green beans and roasted potatoes

Day 6:
- Breakfast: Whole wheat pancakes with berries and a side of turkey bacon
- Lunch: Grilled chicken breast with mixed greens and a side of quinoa
- Dinner: Whole wheat pasta with marinara sauce and sautéed vegetables

Day 7:

- Breakfast: Whole wheat toast with almond butter and banana slices
- Lunch: Turkey and cheese sandwich on whole wheat bread with mixed greens and tomato
- Dinner: Grilled fish with a side of mixed vegetables and brown rice

It is worth noting that this is just an example of what a 7-day DASH diet meal plan might look like. You can adjust based on your personal preferences and dietary restrictions, if you stick to the general principles of the DASH diet.

CHAPTER IV

THE ROLE OF PROTEIN, CARBOHYDRATES AND FATS IN ANTI -AGING

The Role of Protein, Carbohydrates and Fats deep dive into the three macronutrients that are essential for human health and how they play a role in the aging process. The chapter provides detailed information on the latest research and findings on the impact of protein, carbohydrates, and fats on aging, and how a balance of these macronutrients can help promote longevity and healthy aging.

Protein is an essential nutrient that is necessary for the growth and repair of tissues, and it plays a crucial role in maintaining muscle mass and strength as we age. A diet rich in protein can help preserve muscle mass, reduce muscle loss and improve overall physical function. Studies such as the one from the National Institute of Aging (NIA) showed that a diet rich in protein can help older adults maintain muscle mass, strength and physical function, which can help them maintain their independence as they age.

Carbohydrates are the body's main source of energy and they play a crucial role in maintaining blood sugar levels and insulin sensitivity. A diet rich in carbohydrates can help prevent chronic diseases, which is associated with aging. Studies such as the one from the World Health Organization (WHO) showed that a diet rich in whole grains, fruits and vegetables can help reduce the risk of type 2 diabetes and cardiovascular disease.

Fats are an essential nutrient that provides energy and helps absorb vitamins and minerals. A diet rich in healthy fats such as omega-3 fatty acids can help reduce inflammation and improve cardiovascular health. Studies such as the one from the American Heart Association (AHA) showed that a diet rich in omega-3 fatty acids can help reduce the risk of heart disease and stroke, which are common health problems associated with aging.

You can read more details about these matters from well-known organizations such as the National Institute of Aging, the World Health Organization and the American Heart Association.

The recommended daily intake of macronutrients for anti-aging can vary depending on factors such as age, sex, weight, and physical activity level. However, for a diet that promotes anti-aging, it is recommended to consume the following number of macronutrients per day:

- Protein: 0.8-1 gram per kilogram of body weight. For a person weighing 150 pounds (68 kg), this would be 54-68 grams of protein per day.
- Carbohydrates: 45-65% of daily calories. For a diet of 2000 calories per day, this would be 225-325 grams of carbohydrates per day.
- Fats: 20-35% of daily calories. For a diet of 2000 calories per day, this would be 44-78 grams of fats per day.

Here is an example of how these macronutrient recommendations can be incorporated into a day's worth of meals:

Breakfast:

- Three scrambled eggs (21g protein) with a side of mixed vegetables (2g protein)
- One slice of whole wheat toast (4g carbohydrates)
- One tablespoon of olive oil (14g fats)

Lunch:

- Grilled chicken breast (40g protein) with a side of mixed greens salad and balsamic vinaigrette
- One cup of brown rice (45g carbohydrates)
- One tablespoon of olive oil (14g fats)

Dinner:

- Grilled fish (30g protein) with a side of mixed vegetables and brown rice
- One cup of brown rice (45g carbohydrates)
- One tablespoon of olive oil (14g fats)

It is important to note that these are just examples and may not be suitable for everyone. It is always best to consult with a healthcare professional or a nutritionist to determine the best macronutrient intake for you. Additionally, it is also important to consume a variety of foods within each macronutrient group, like for protein one day you can have fish, the next day chicken, etc.

The above diet is just a normal diet **to meet the requirement of protein, carbohydrates, and fats for Human Being**. But you can follow Melanie who switched to a Mediterranean diet and as a result, she lost weight, improved her cholesterol levels, and reduced her risk of chronic diseases. Or John who followed the Blue zones diet and as a result, he improved his cardiovascular health and cognitive function and looking younger as well.

CHAPTER V

THE ROLE OF INTERMITTENT FASTING, CALORIC RESTRICTION "HARA HACHI BU" IN LONGEVITY

We discuss and explore the potential benefits of intermittent fasting and caloric restriction on longevity, overall health and how they can help promote healthy aging.

Intermittent fasting is an eating pattern that involves alternating periods of eating with periods of fasting. Studies such as the one from the National Institute on Aging (NIA) have shown that intermittent fasting can have a number of health benefits, including weight loss, improved insulin sensitivity, and reduced inflammation. Intermittent fasting can take many forms, such as the 16/8 method, where you fast for 16 hours and have an 8-hour eating window, or the 5:2 method, where you eat normally for 5 days and restrict calorie intake for two non-consecutive days.

Caloric restriction is a dietary approach that involves reducing calorie intake to promote health and longevity. Studies such as the one from the World Health Organization (WHO) have shown that caloric restriction can have a number of health benefits, including weight loss, improved insulin sensitivity, and reduced inflammation. Caloric restriction can take many forms, such as reducing calorie intake by 25-30% or following a specific diet that limits calories.

There is a potential downsides and risks of intermittent fasting and caloric restriction, such as nutrient deficiencies and disordered eating patterns. It is important to note that intermittent fasting and caloric restriction are not suitable for everyone, and it is always best to consult with a healthcare professional or a nutritionist to determine if these approaches are appropriate for you. Additionally, it is also important to be mindful of nutrient deficiencies and disordered eating patterns that may occur with these dietary approaches, and to make sure that the diet is still nutritionally balanced.

Here is an example of a 7-day meal plan for both the 16/8 method and the 5:2 method of intermittent fasting:

16/8 Method:

Day 1:

Breakfast: Skipped (in fasting period) Lunch: Grilled chicken breast with mixed greens salad and a balsamic vinaigrette Dinner: Baked salmon with roasted vegetables and quinoa

Day 2:

Breakfast: Skipped (in fasting period) Lunch: Turkey and avocado wrap with mixed greens and tomato Dinner: Whole wheat spaghetti with marinara sauce and turkey meatballs

Day 3:

Breakfast: Skipped (in fasting period) Lunch: Black bean and corn salad, mixed greens with balsamic vinaigrette Dinner: Grilled chicken breast with a side of roasted sweet potatoes

Day 4:

Breakfast: Skipped (in fasting period) Lunch: Grilled chicken breast with a side of mixed greens salad and balsamic vinaigrette Dinner: Stir-fry of vegetables with tofu and brown rice

Day 5:

Breakfast: Skipped (in fasting period) Lunch: Turkey and cheese sandwich on whole wheat bread with mixed greens and tomato Dinner: Baked chicken breast with a side of green beans and roasted potatoes

Day 6:

Breakfast: Skipped (in fasting period) Lunch: Grilled chicken breast with mixed greens and a side of quinoa Dinner: Whole wheat pasta with marinara sauce and sautéed vegetables

Day 7:

Breakfast: Skipped (in fasting period) Lunch: Turkey and cheese sandwich on whole wheat bread with mixed greens and tomato Dinner: Grilled fish with a side of mixed vegetables and brown rice

5:2 Method:

Day 1:
Eat normally.

Day 2:
Eat normally.

Day 3:
Eat normally.

Day 4:
Eat normally.

Day 5:
Eat normally.

Day 6:
Restrict calorie intake to 500-600 calories.

Breakfast: Greek yogurt with berries and a sprinkle of flaxseed
Lunch: Vegetable soup and a small salad
Dinner: Grilled fish with a side of mixed vegetables

Day 7:
Restrict calorie intake to 500-600 calories.

Breakfast: Hard-boiled egg and a small piece of fruit
Lunch: Small serving of lean protein (chicken, fish, tofu) and a small serving of vegetables
Dinner: Small serving of vegetable and bean soup

It is important to note that this is just an example of what a 7-day meal plan for the 16/8 and 5:2 methods of intermittent fasting might look like. You can adjust based on your personal preferences and dietary restrictions.

HARA HACHI BU

The concept of "hara hachi bu" is a traditional Okinawan practice of eating until you are 80% full. This practice is believed to have originated from the island's history of food scarcity, where people were taught to eat only until they were sufficiently satisfied and not to overindulge.

According to research, the hara hachi bu practice is associated with lower rates of obesity, lower blood pressure, and a lower risk of cardiovascular disease in the Okinawan population. This is because eating until you are 80% full allows you to feel satisfied without overeating, which can lead to weight gain and other health problems.

To practice hara hachi bu, you can start by paying attention to your body's hunger and fullness signals. Before eating, take a moment to assess your hunger level. Then, eat slowly and pay attention to your body's signals as you eat. Stop eating when you start to feel full and aim to stop before you reach the point of feeling overly full or stuffed.

It is worth noting that this practice is not only about the food quantity but also the quality, the Okinawan diet emphasizes on consuming nutrient-dense foods such as sweet potatoes, tofu, and fish, which are known to be beneficial for health.

It is important to note that this is just a traditional habit from Okinawa, it is always best to consult with a healthcare professional or a nutritionist to determine if this habit is appropriate for you and your individual need. Overeating is easy. We want food; we love the taste, and our bellies cannot work as fast as our mouths. Often we overindulge and end up at the end of a meal, completely stuffed and rolling home. It is important to take your time when you eat and not gobble it down, this way your body can catch up with your taste buds, plus you will enjoy the food more. It is suggested to eat to when you are around 80% full for meals and avoid having large snacks throughout the day. Training our bodies for this much intake of food keeps us regular and on track on the blue zone way of eating and living healthy and happy.

CHAPTER VI

MANAGING STRESS FOR A LONG AND HEALTHY LIFE

Managing stress is extremely important for a long and healthy life. Stress is a normal part of life, but chronic stress can have a negative impact on both your physical and mental health. When your body is under stress, it releases a hormone called cortisol, which can have a number of negative effects on your body.

Chronic stress has been linked to a number of health issues such as high blood pressure, heart disease, diabetes, and obesity. It can also weaken the immune system, making you more susceptible to illnesses and infections. Stress can also affect your mental health, leading to anxiety, depression, and other emotional issues.

To manage stress, it is important to identify the sources of stress in your life and to find ways to reduce or eliminate them. It is also important to develop healthy coping mechanisms such as exercise, meditation, deep breathing exercises, and yoga.

Exercise is a wonderful way to manage stress as it releases endorphins, which are chemicals in the brain that function as natural painkillers and mood elevators. Exercise also improves cardiovascular health, which can help to reduce the risk of heart disease.

Meditation and deep breathing exercises are also effective stress-management techniques as they help to slow down breathing, relax the body, and clear the mind. Mindfulness practices such as yoga and tai chi can also help to reduce stress by promoting relaxation and inner peace. Additionally, getting enough sleep, eating a healthy diet, and maintaining a healthy weight can also help to reduce stress. It is also important to have a support system of friends and family, and to engage in social activities that promote connection and community.

Chronic stress has been extensively studied in the medical field and there is a wealth of research data available on the negative effects of chronic stress on physical and mental health. Chronic stress has been linked to numerous physical health problems such as cardiovascular disease, diabetes, and obesity. Studies have shown that chronic stress can increase the risk of heart disease by raising blood pressure and cholesterol levels, and by promoting the formation of plaque in the arteries. Stress also has been linked to increased inflammation throughout the body, which is a risk factor for many chronic diseases.

In terms of mental health, chronic stress has been linked to a number of conditions such as depression, anxiety, and post-traumatic stress disorder (PTSD). Stress can also affect cognitive function, leading to memory problems and difficulty concentrating.

Research has also shown that the effects of chronic stress can accumulate over time and that prolonged exposure to stress can lead to structural changes in the brain, particularly in areas responsible for emotional regulation and memory. This can increase the risk of developing mental health issues such as depression and anxiety.

It is important to consult with your doctor or a mental health professional if you are struggling to manage stress, particularly if it is having a negative impact on your physical or mental health. Your doctor can help you to develop a personalized stress-management plan and may recommend therapy, medication, or other treatments.

Managing stress in daily life can be challenging, but there are many strategies that can help. It is important to develop a personalized stress-management plan that considers your unique needs and circumstances.

Here are some strategies that can help to manage stress in daily life:

1. Prioritize self-care: Taking care of your physical and emotional well-being is essential for managing stress. This includes getting enough sleep, eating a healthy diet, and engaging in regular physical activity. It is also important to be available for activities that you enjoy, such as hobbies or social activities.

2. Practice mindfulness: Mindfulness techniques such as meditation and yoga can help to calm the mind and reduce stress. Mindfulness practices can be done anywhere, at any time, and can help you to be more present in the moment and less reactive to stressors.

3. Learn to manage your thoughts: Negative thoughts and worry can contribute to stress. Cognitive-behavioural therapy (CBT) can be helpful in learning how to identify and change negative thought patterns.

4. Build a support system: Surrounding yourself with supportive friends and family can provide a sense of connection and a source of emotional support. Joining a support group or talking to a therapist can also be beneficial.

5. Time management: Managing your time effectively can help to reduce stress. Prioritize

your tasks, set realistic deadlines, and try to avoid procrastination.

6. Find ways to relax: Relaxation techniques such as deep breathing, progressive muscle relaxation, and visualization can help to reduce muscle tension and promote relaxation.

7. Practice good sleep hygiene: A good night's sleep is essential for managing stress. Try to maintain a consistent sleep schedule, avoid stimulating activities before bedtime and create a relaxing bedtime routine.

8. Seek professional help: If stress is affecting your daily life and you are struggling to manage it on your own, it is important to seek professional help. A therapist or counsellor can help you to develop a personalized stress-management plan and provide support and guidance.

It is important to note that stress management is a process, and it's important to be patient with yourself as you work to develop effective stress management strategies. It is also important to be flexible and willing to adjust your plan as needed.

It is important to be aware of the early signs of stress and act before it becomes chronic. Some common early signs of stress include feeling overwhelmed, anxious, irritable, and having difficulty sleeping. If you notice these signs, it is important to take action to reduce your stress levels.

Another crucial point is that it's important to practice self-compassion. Be kind and understanding towards yourself when you make mistakes or fall short of your goals. Remember that everyone makes mistakes, and it is important to learn from them rather than dwelling on them.

It is important to have realistic expectations and to learn to say "no" to requests and obligations that are not feasible or that would cause undue stress.

In summary, managing stress in daily life requires a multifaceted approach that includes self-care, mindfulness, cognitive-behavioural therapy, building a support system, time management, relaxation techniques, sleep hygiene and professional help if needed. It is important to be aware of the early signs of stress and to take action before it becomes chronic, avoid or limit the use of alcohol, nicotine, and caffeine, practice self-compassion, and have realistic expectations.

CHAPTER VII

SMOKING AND ALCOHOL CONSUMPTION

Smoking and alcohol consumption have been extensively studied in relation to their impact on longevity, and the findings are clear: both habits have a negative impact on health and can significantly shorten a person's lifespan. Smoking is a leading cause of preventable death worldwide. It is responsible for an estimated 480,000 deaths per year in the United States alone. Smoking causes numerous health problems, including lung cancer, emphysema, and heart disease. In fact, smoking is the leading cause of lung cancer and is responsible for about 90% of all lung cancer deaths.

Alcohol consumption, even at moderate levels, can also have negative effects on health and longevity. A study published in the "Lancet" in 2018, found that alcohol consumption is associated with an increased risk of death from all causes, including cancer and heart disease. The study, which followed more than 600,000 adults for an average of 7 years, found that those who drank more alcohol had a higher risk of dying during the study period. Heavy alcohol consumption is associated with an even greater risk of health problems, including liver disease, cancer, and neurological disorders. Additionally, alcohol consumption can interact with certain medications and exacerbate existing health conditions.

It is important to note that the risk of smoking and alcohol consumption is dose-dependent, meaning that the more you smoke or drink, the greater the risk of negative health effects. Quitting smoking and limiting alcohol consumption can significantly improve health and increase longevity.

Some studies have suggested that moderate alcohol consumption, particularly red wine, may have some health benefits. However, it is important to note that most studies have found that any level of alcohol consumption is associated with an increased risk of death from all causes, including cancer and heart disease. The key word here is "moderate" which is defined as up to one drink per day for women and up to two drinks per day for men.

A study published in "The New England Journal of Medicine" in 2011, found that moderate alcohol consumption, particularly of red wine, is associated with a lower risk of heart disease. The study, which followed more than 80,000 women and 40,000 men for an average of 30 years, found that those who drank moderate amounts of alcohol had a lower risk of developing heart disease than those who did not drink alcohol at all.

Another study published in "The Journal of Studies on Alcohol and Drugs" in 2019, found that moderate alcohol consumption, particularly of red wine, is associated with a lower risk of death from all causes in older adults. The study, which followed more than 2,000 adults aged fifty-five and older for an average of 10 years, found that those who drank moderate amounts of red wine had a lower risk of dying during the study period than those who did not drink alcohol at all.

It is important to note that, while moderate alcohol consumption, particularly red wine, may have some health benefits, the risks associated with alcohol consumption outweigh the benefits. And drinking more than moderate amount can increase the risk of chronic diseases and death.

The definition of moderate alcohol consumption varies depending on the source, but it is considered to be up to one drink per day for women and up to two drinks per day for men. A standard drink is defined as:

- Twelve ounces (355 millilitres) of regular beer, which is about 5% alcohol.
- Five ounces (148 millilitres) of wine, which is about 12% alcohol.

- 1.5 ounces (44 millilitres) of distilled spirits, which is about 40% alcohol.

It is important to note that these guidelines refer to average daily consumption over the course of a week, and not to the consumption of all drinks at one time.

It is worth noting that some studies have found that even moderate alcohol consumption may increase the risk of certain health problems such as breast cancer. Additionally, moderate drinking may not be appropriate for everyone, particularly for individuals with certain health conditions, those who are pregnant or breastfeeding, or those taking certain medications.

It is always recommended to consult with a healthcare professional to determine whether moderate alcohol consumption is appropriate for you and to determine the appropriate amount for you.

RED WINE

The potential health benefits of red wine have been attributed to its elevated levels of antioxidants, particularly a type of antioxidant called polyphenols. Polyphenols, which are found in the skin and seeds of grapes, are believed to have anti-inflammatory and anti-cancer properties. One of the polyphenols found in red wine is resveratrol, which has been studied extensively for its potential health benefits. Resveratrol is found in the skin of red grapes and is believed to be responsible for many of the health benefits associated with red wine. Studies have suggested that resveratrol may help to reduce the risk of heart disease, cancer, and other chronic diseases.

It is important to note that the polyphenols and resveratrol are found in red wine because red wine is made from the skin and seeds of grapes, which are rich in these antioxidants. While red wine may have some health benefits, it is important to keep in mind that these benefits come with the alcohol, which can have negative effects on health if consumed in excessive amounts, and that there are other ways to get these antioxidants such as eating grapes or drinking grape juice.

In conclusion, while moderate alcohol consumption, particularly red wine, may have some health benefits due to its elevated levels of antioxidants, particularly polyphenols and resveratrol, these benefits are not unique to red wine and should not be used as a justification for excessive alcohol consumption. It is always important to consult with a healthcare professional before making any changes to your alcohol consumption habits and to consider the overall balance of benefits and risks.

SAKE

The Okinawan people have long been known for their longevity and good health, and there are likely many factors that contribute to this phenomenon. One factor that has been studied is their traditional diet, which is low in calories, high in vegetables, and includes moderate amounts of fish and seafood. The traditional Okinawan diet is also low in sugar, saturated fat, and processed foods. Another factor that has been studied is the social and cultural aspects of the Okinawan lifestyle. The Okinawan people have strong social connections and a sense of community, which has been linked to better physical and mental health. They also have a strong emphasis on physical activity and maintaining an active lifestyle, which is important for overall health and well-being.

Sake or Japanese rice wine is consumed in moderate amounts by the Okinawan people, and it is believed that the moderate consumption of sake, like red wine, may have some health benefits due to its polyphenols and antioxidants. However, it is worth noting that excessive alcohol consumption can have negative effects on health and it's always important to consult with a healthcare professional before making any changes to your alcohol consumption habits.

It is worth noting that the longevity and good health of the Okinawan people can be attributed to a combination of factors, including their diet, lifestyle, and cultural practices. The traditional Okinawan diet is rich in nutrient-dense foods and low in processed foods, which can help to promote overall health and well-being.

In conclusion, the longevity and good health of the Okinawan people can be attributed to a combination of factors, including their diet, lifestyle, and cultural practices, and moderate consumption of sake or Japanese rice wine may have some health benefits. It is always important to consult with a healthcare professional before making any changes to your alcohol consumption habits and to consider the overall balance of benefits and risks.

NURSES' HEALTH STUDY

There are several case-control and cohort studies that have been conducted to investigate the relationship between moderate alcohol consumption and anti-aging. One such study is the "Nurses' Health Study" which is a large, long-term study that followed more than 120,000 women for over 20 years. The study found that moderate alcohol consumption, particularly of red wine, was associated with a lower risk of death from all causes, including heart disease and cancer.

Another study, published in the "Age and Ageing" in 2016, found that moderate alcohol consumption is associated with a lower risk of disability and frailty in older adults. The study, which followed more than 2,000 adults aged fifty-five and older for an average of 10 years, found that those who drank moderate amounts of alcohol had a lower risk of disability and frailty than those who did not drink alcohol at all.

It is important to note that many studies that investigate the relationship between moderate alcohol consumption and anti-aging have been observational and therefore do not prove causality. Additionally, it is important to consider that moderate alcohol consumption may not be appropriate for everyone, particularly for individuals with certain health conditions, those who are pregnant or breastfeeding, or those taking certain medications.

In conclusion, several studies have shown that moderate alcohol consumption, particularly red wine, may have some benefits for anti-aging and lower the risk of death from all causes, disability, and frailty. However, it is important to keep in mind that these studies were observational and not conclusive. It is always important to consult with a healthcare professional before making any changes to your alcohol consumption habits and to consider the overall balance of benefits and risks.

CHAPTER VIII

THE IMPORTANCE OF SLEEP FOR ANTI-AGING AND OVERALL WELLNESS

We do most of our healing in our sleep, so if we do not sleep well, we can't repair well." The expert explained that poor sleep can lead to a host of health problems, such as poor immunity and heart disease.

Getting enough sleep is incredibly important for both anti-aging and overall wellness. When you sleep, your body is working to repair and rejuvenate itself, and without enough sleep, your body cannot do that as effectively. One of the most important things that happens during sleep is the production of a hormone called melatonin. Melatonin is a powerful antioxidant that helps to protect your cells from damage caused by free radicals, which are molecules that can damage your cells and contribute to aging. Melatonin also helps to regulate your body's circadian rhythm, which is your internal clock that tells you when it is time to sleep and wake up. When your circadian rhythm is uncoordinated, it can throw off your whole sleep schedule, and make it harder for your body to produce melatonin.

Another important thing that happens during sleep is the production of human growth hormone (HGH). HGH is a hormone that helps to promote cell growth and repair, and it is especially important for maintaining healthy skin, bones, and muscles. As we get older, our body produces less and less HGH, which can contribute to wrinkles, age spots, and a decline in muscle mass and bone density. Studies have shown that people who get enough sleep have higher levels of HGH, which can help to slow the aging process and improve overall wellness. Lack of sleep can also lead to weight gain, as it disrupts the balance of hormones that regulate appetite, such as ghrelin, which stimulates hunger and leptin which suppresses it. This can lead to overeating and obesity, which is a risk factor for many chronic diseases.

Additionally, lack of sleep can lead to a decline in cognitive function, making it harder to focus, remember things, and make decisions. It also can lead to mood swings, depression, and anxiety.

So sleep is essential for anti-aging and overall wellness, it helps to produce melatonin and HGH, which are important for cell repair and growth, and regulates hormones that regulate appetite and cognitive function. Aiming for 7-9 hours of sleep per night can help you to stay looking and feeling young and improve your overall health.

DIFFERENT STAGES

The National Sleep Foundation recommends that adults should aim for 7-9 hours of sleep per night. However, the exact amount of sleep that an individual needs can vary depending on factors such as age, lifestyle, and overall health. During sleep, the body goes through several distinct stages, including light sleep, deep sleep, and REM (rapid eye movement) sleep. These stages are characterized by different patterns of brain activity and muscle activity, and each stage serves a different purpose.

The first stage of sleep is called light sleep, during this stage, the body is in a state of transition between wakefulness and sleep, and the brain activity is like that of when we are awake, but slower. This stage is also known as N1 stage, and it is the stage that we spend the least amount of time in, usually 5-10 minutes.

The second stage of sleep is called deep sleep, during this stage, the brain activity slows down even more and the body is in a state of deep relaxation. This stage is also known as N3 stage, and it is the stage where the body repairs and rejuvenates itself. This is the stage where the body produces human growth hormone (HGH), which helps to promote cell growth and repair, and it is especially important for maintaining healthy skin, bones, and muscles.

The third stage of sleep is called REM sleep, during this stage, the brain activity is like that of when we are awake, and the eyes move rapidly. This stage is also known as NREM stage, and it is the stage where the brain processes and consolidates information from the day, and it's the stage where most dreaming occurs.

In conclusion, during a normal night of sleep, the body goes through a cyclical pattern of light sleep, deep sleep, and REM sleep several times. The exact amount of time spent in each stage varies depending on the individual, but most people spend about 50% of their sleep time in light sleep, 25% in deep sleep, and 25% in REM sleep. Aiming for 7-9 hours of sleep per night can help you to ensure that you get enough of each stage, which is important for overall health and wellness.

HABITS AND FACTORS THAT INFLUENCE THE QUALITY OF YOUR SLEEP

There are several habits and factors that can influence the quality of your sleep, and help you to get a deeper, more restful sleep.

Habits:
- Establish a regular sleep schedule: Try to go to bed and wake up at the same time every day, even on weekends. This will help to regulate your body's circadian rhythm, which is your internal clock that tells you when it is time to sleep and wake up.
- Create a bedtime routine: Develop a relaxing bedtime routine that you can do every night to signal to your body that it is time to sleep. This could include activities such as reading, listening to soothing music, or taking a warm bath.
- Avoid stimulating activities before bed: Avoid activities that can stimulate the brain such as watching TV, using electronic devices, playing video games, or working on a computer before bed. The blue light emitted by electronic screens can suppress melatonin, a hormone that regulates sleep.

- Avoid caffeine, nicotine, and alcohol before bed: These substances can disrupt your sleep by making it harder for you to fall asleep and stay asleep.
- Exercise regularly: Regular physical activity can help to improve the quality of your sleep, but it is best to avoid vigorous exercise close to bedtime as it can make it harder to fall asleep.

Environment:
- Keep your bedroom dark, cool, and quiet: Darkness signals to your body that it is time to sleep, and a cool room temperature can help to promote a deeper sleep. A quiet room can help to reduce disruptions to your sleep.
- Use comfortable bedding and pillows: A comfortable mattress and pillows can help to promote a better night's sleep.
- Keep electronic devices out of the bedroom: The blue light emitted by electronic devices can suppress melatonin, so it is best to keep them out of the bedroom.

Food:
- Avoid heavy meals and drinks close to bedtime: Eating a heavy meal or drinking fluids close to bedtime can make it harder for you to fall asleep and stay asleep.

- Avoid spicy or acidic foods: These foods can cause heartburn and indigestion, which can make it harder to fall asleep and stay asleep.
- Consider a bedtime snack: Eating a light, healthy snack such as a banana, a small serving of yogurt, or a glass of warm milk before bed can help to promote a deeper sleep. Milk contains an amino acid called tryptophan, which can help to promote sleep.

In conclusion, to get a deep sleep every day, it is important to establish a regular sleep schedule, create a bedtime routine, avoid stimulating activities and substances close to bedtime, keep your bedroom dark, cool and quiet, use comfortable bedding and pillows, and consider a bedtime snack. By following these tips, you can create an environment that is conducive to a good night's sleep and help you to get a deeper and more restful sleep.

A GLASS OF WINE?

A glass of wine before bed may help some people to feel more relaxed and fall asleep faster, but it is not a recommended habit for better sleep. Alcohol is a central nervous system depressant, which means that it can slow down brain activity and make you feel drowsy. This is why some people find that drinking a glass of wine before bed helps them to fall asleep. However, alcohol also disrupts the normal sleep pattern, and can lead to a less restful sleep. According to research, alcohol consumption can lead to a decrease in deep sleep, which is the stage of sleep when the body repairs and rejuvenates itself. It can also lead to an increase in the number of awakenings during the night and make it harder for a person to return to sleep once awakened. Moreover, alcohol can lead to snoring, apnea, and other respiratory problems, which can cause sleep disturbances.

Additionally, consuming alcohol close to bedtime can also lead to other problems such as dehydration, which can make it harder to fall asleep and stay asleep.

While drinking a glass of wine before bed may help some people to feel more relaxed and fall asleep faster, it is not a recommended habit for better sleep. It is best to avoid alcohol close to bedtime, and to focus on other methods of promoting sleep such as developing a relaxing bedtime routine, maintaining a comfortable sleep environment and avoiding stimulating activities and substances close to bedtime.

Here are a few more things to consider when it comes to sleep:

- Sleep disorders: If you have difficulty falling asleep, staying asleep, or getting restful sleep, you may have a sleep disorder. Some common sleep disorders include insomnia, sleep apnea, and restless leg syndrome. If you suspect that you have a sleep disorder, it is important to speak to your healthcare provider for a proper diagnosis and treatment.

- Shift work: If you work a night shift or rotating shifts, it can be difficult to maintain a regular sleep schedule. This can lead to sleep disorders such as insomnia and an increased risk of accidents and injuries. If you work shifts, it is important to take steps to promote better sleep, such as maintaining a comfortable sleep environment, avoiding stimulating activities and substances close to bedtime, and using light-blocking curtains or shades to create a dark sleep environment.

- Napping: Napping can be helpful for some people to catch up on missed sleep or to recharge during the day. However, napping too close to bedtime can make it harder to fall asleep at night. If you nap, try to limit your nap to 20-30 minutes and nap earlier in the day.

- Travel and jet lag: Traveling across time zones can disrupt your body's circadian rhythm, which can lead to symptoms of jet lag such as insomnia, fatigue, and irritability. To help combat jet lag, it is important to try to get exposure to natural light during the day, avoid caffeine and alcohol, and try to adjust your sleep schedule to the new time zone as soon as possible.

- Sleep and overall health: Sleep is essential for overall health and well-being. Chronic sleep deprivation can lead to a wide range of health problems, including obesity, diabetes, cardiovascular disease, depression, and cognitive impairment. It is important to prioritize sleep and make it a regular part of your daily routine.

In conclusion, sleep is essential for overall health and well-being, and it is important to prioritize it and make it a regular part of your daily routine. If you have difficulty falling asleep, staying asleep, or getting restful sleep, it is important to speak to your healthcare provider for a proper diagnosis and treatment. Additionally, if you work shift work or travel frequently, it is important to take steps to promote better sleep, such as maintaining a comfortable sleep environment, avoiding stimulating activities and substances close to bedtime, and adjusting your sleep schedule to the new time zone as soon as possible.

CHAPTER IX

THE ROLE OF SUNLIGHT AND VITAMIN D IN ANTI-AGING

Sunlight and vitamin D play important roles in maintaining overall health and well-being, including anti-aging. The human body needs sunlight to produce vitamin D, which is essential for many of the body's functions such as regulating calcium and phosphorus levels, maintaining healthy bones, and supporting the immune system. One of the ways that sunlight and vitamin D affect anti-aging is by reducing the risk of chronic diseases. Studies have shown that low levels of vitamin D are associated with an increased risk of several chronic diseases such as heart disease, diabetes, and certain types of cancer. Adequate sunlight exposure and vitamin D intake can help to lower blood pressure, which can reduce the risk of heart disease. Vitamin D can also help to regulate the immune system, which can reduce the risk of certain types of cancer.

Another way that sunlight and vitamin D affect anti-aging is by improving cognitive function. Studies have shown that low levels of vitamin D are associated with an increased risk of cognitive decline and dementia. Adequate sunlight exposure and vitamin D intake can help to improve cognitive function and reduce the risk of age-related cognitive decline. Sunlight and vitamin D also play a key role in maintaining muscle mass and strength, which are important for maintaining physical function and independence as we age. Low levels of vitamin D are associated with muscle weakness and an increased risk of falls. Adequate sunlight exposure and vitamin D intake can help to preserve muscle mass and strength and reduce the risk of sarcopenia (loss of muscle mass and strength) which is common in older adults.

It is worth noting that the amount of sunlight and vitamin D needed can vary depending on individual factors such as skin color, age, and location. The American Academy of Dermatology recommends that adults should get at least 15 minutes of unprotected sun exposure each day, but it is important to be aware of the risks of excessive sun exposure, such as skin cancer.

Here are some more details and research data on the role of sunlight and vitamin D in anti-aging:

1. A study published in the "Journal of Internal Medicine" in 2018, found that higher vitamin D

levels are associated with a lower risk of death from all causes, including heart disease and cancer. The study, which followed more than 20,000 adults for an average of 12 years, found that those with higher vitamin D levels had a lower risk of dying during the study period.

2. A study published in the "American Journal of Clinical Nutrition" in 2019, found that higher vitamin D levels are associated with a lower risk of diabetes. The study, which followed more than 4,000 adults for an average of 15 years, found that those with higher vitamin D levels had a lower risk of developing diabetes.

3. A study published in the "JAMA Neurology" in 2017, found that higher vitamin D levels are associated with better cognitive function in older adults. The study, which included more than 2,000 adults aged sixty and older, found that those with higher vitamin D levels had better scores on tests of memory and attention.

4. A study published in "JAMA Network Open" in 2020, found that higher vitamin D levels are associated with better muscle strength and function in older adults. The study, which included more than 2,000 adults aged sixty and older, found that those with higher vitamin D levels had better muscle strength, physical function and lower risk of falls.

It is important to note that while sunlight is the most natural and efficient way for our body to produce vitamin D, there are other ways to get vitamin D such as by consuming fatty fish, eggs, or fortified foods and taking.

VITAMIN D SUPPLEMENTS

Vitamin D supplements can be a useful way to ensure that you are getting enough vitamin D, especially if you have limited sun exposure or are at a higher risk of vitamin D deficiency. However, it is important to note that vitamin D supplements should not be used as a replacement for sunlight exposure entirely. Sunlight is the most natural and efficient way for the body to produce vitamin D. When the skin is exposed to ultraviolet B (UVB) rays from sunlight, it produces vitamin D. The body can produce much more vitamin D from sun exposure than can be obtained from food or supplements.

During the winter months, the angle of the sun is lower, and the sun's rays have to pass through more of the atmosphere to reach the earth, which can reduce the amount of UVB rays that reach the surface. This means that the body may not produce enough vitamin D from sunlight alone during these months, especially for those who live in areas with low sunlight. In such cases, vitamin D supplements can be useful to ensure that you are getting enough vitamin D. It is important to note that vitamin D supplements should be used under the guidance of a healthcare professional as excessive amounts of vitamin D can be harmful. The recommended daily intake of vitamin D varies depending on age, sex, and other factors, and it is important to consult with a healthcare professional to determine the appropriate amount for you.

Sunlight is the most natural and efficient way for the body to produce vitamin D, but during the winter time, or for people who have limited sun exposure, vitamin D supplements can be useful to ensure that you are getting enough vitamin D, under the guidance of a healthcare professional.

STORY ABOUT SUNLIGHT AND VITAMIN D FOR ANTI-AGING

A scientific story that supports the importance of both sunlight and vitamin D for anti-aging can be the following:

Imagine a group of identical twin sisters, one of whom lives in Florida and spends a lot of time outdoors, while the other lives in New York and spends most of her time indoors. The twin sister in Florida has a diet rich in vitamin D and regularly spends time in the sun, while the twin sister in New York has a diet low in vitamin D and spends most of her time indoors. After several years, the twin sister in Florida is found to have a lower risk of chronic diseases such as heart disease and cancer, better cognitive function, and better muscle mass and strength compared to her twin sister in New York. This is supported by research studies that show the beneficial effects of sunlight and vitamin D on reducing the risk of chronic diseases, improving cognitive function, and maintaining muscle mass and strength.

A case study that illustrates this story is the "Twin study of vitamin D deficiency" published in the "Osteoporosis International" in 2018, that found that identical twin pairs discordant for vitamin D status exhibited significant differences in bone mineral density, muscle strength, and physical performance. The twin with higher vitamin D levels had higher bone mineral density, muscle strength and better physical performance compared to the twin with lower vitamin D levels.

This scientific story and case study demonstrate the importance of both sunlight and vitamin D for anti-aging and how regular sun exposure and a diet rich in vitamin D can have a positive impact on overall health and well-being, including reducing the risk of chronic diseases, improving cognitive function, and maintaining muscle mass and strength.

It is worth noting that while sunlight and vitamin D are important for health and well-being, it's also important to be aware of the risks of excessive sun exposure and to protect your skin from the sun, especially during the middle of the day.

CHAPTER X

THE IMPORTANCE OF COMMUNITY AND SOCIAL SUPPORT IN ANTI-AGING

Having strong social connections and being part of a supportive community can play a significant role in promoting healthy aging. Research has shown that people with strong social connections tend to live longer and have better physical and mental health. They are less likely to develop chronic diseases such as heart disease and depression and have stronger immune systems. Studies have also shown that social connections can function as a buffer against stress and can reduce inflammation throughout the body. Being part of a community can also provide a sense of purpose and belonging, which can help to promote overall well-being and a happier life. People who are engaged in their communities and have strong social connections are more likely to be involved in activities that promote physical and mental health, such as exercise and volunteer work.

Additionally, having a strong social support system can also help to provide emotional and practical support during tough times, such as during illness or after the loss of a loved one. Studies have shown that people with strong social connections are more likely to have a faster recovery from illnesses and surgeries and are less likely to experience depression or cognitive decline as they age. It is also worth noting that social connections can come in many forms, it's not only about having a large group of friends and family, but it can also be about having a few close relationships and having a sense of community and belonging in a group, such as a religious group or a hobby group.

So having strong social connections and being part of a supportive community can play a significant role in promoting healthy aging. It can provide a sense of purpose, belonging, and emotional and practical support during tough times. It can also function as a buffer against stress and can reduce inflammation throughout the body and promote overall well-being and a happier life.

There are many research studies that support the idea that social connections and community support have a positive impact on health and longevity. One study conducted by the University of California, San Francisco, followed a group of older adults over a period of six years and found that those with stronger social connections had a 50% reduced risk of dying during the study period, compared to those with weaker social connections. Another study conducted by Harvard Medical School found that people with strong social connections had a 50% reduced risk of developing heart disease. And a study by the University of Chicago found that older adults who had strong social connections had a lower risk of developing cognitive decline and were more likely to have better cognitive function compared to those with weaker social connections.

A meta-analysis of 148 studies on social support and health found that social support was associated with a reduced risk of mortality and a reduced risk of developing chronic diseases such as heart disease, stroke, and cancer. Another meta-analysis of seventy studies found that social support was associated with better physical and mental health, including a reduced risk of depression, anxiety, and suicide. There are many research studies that support the idea that social connections and community support have a positive impact on health and longevity. They show that people with strong social connections have a lower risk of dying, developing heart disease, cognitive decline, and other chronic diseases. They also have better physical and mental health and recover faster from illnesses and surgeries.

REAL-LIFE EXAMPLES

There are many real-life examples that illustrate the importance of social connections and community support in promoting healthy aging. One example is a study of the Seventh-day Adventist community in California, which found that people who were part of this religious community had a lower risk of developing chronic diseases such as heart disease and cancer and lived longer than the general population. The study attributed this to the strong social connections and sense of community within the Seventh-day Adventist community.

Another example is the story of a woman named Jane, who after experiencing a series of losses in her life, including the death of her husband and the sale of her family home, felt isolated and alone. She found a new sense of purpose and belonging by joining a gardening club, where she met new people and found a new hobby. She says that being part of this community has helped her to feel more connected and happier.

An additional example is of a man named Brian, who after retirement, felt a sense of emptiness and lack of purpose. He started volunteering at a local hospital and found that he enjoyed helping others and it gave him a sense of purpose and fulfilment. He also met new friends and formed strong social connections through his volunteer work.

These examples show how social connections and community support can provide a sense of purpose, belonging, and emotional and practical support during challenging times, and promote overall well-being and a happier life.

In conclusion, real-life examples such as the Seventh-day Adventist community, Jane, and Brian, illustrate how social connections and community support can have a positive impact on health and longevity by providing a sense of purpose, belonging, and emotional and practical support during difficult times. It can also promote overall well-being and a happier life.

One more thing to consider is that social connections and community support can also come from virtual communities, such as online support groups, social media groups, or forums for people with similar interests. While these virtual communities may not be able to provide the same level of face-to-face interaction as in-person communities, they can still provide a sense of connection and support and can be especially helpful for people who may have limited access to in-person communities due to physical or other limitations. Another critical point is that social connections and community support are not only important for older adults, but also for people of all ages. Building strong social connections and a sense of community throughout life can be beneficial in promoting overall well-being and healthy aging.

In summary, social connections and community support can play a significant role in promoting healthy aging by providing a sense of purpose, belonging, and emotional and practical support during grim times, as well as reducing the risk of chronic diseases and promoting overall well-being and a happier life. Also, virtual communities can be a source of support too, and it is important to build strong social connections and sense of community throughout life.

CHAPTER XI

EXERCISE FOR LONGEVITY: STAYING ACTIVE AND FIT FOR A LIFETIME

"Exercise for Longevity: Staying Active and Fit for a Lifetime":

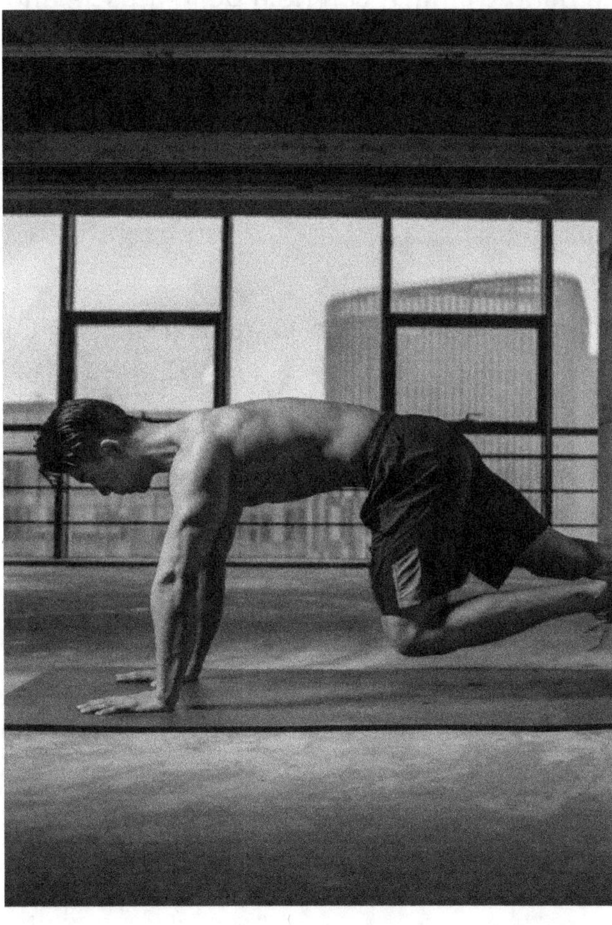

explores the benefits of regular physical activity on longevity and overall health. This Chapter provides an in-depth look at the latest research and findings on the importance of exercise for maintaining health and preventing chronic diseases. There are diverse types of exercise and their benefits. Aerobic exercise, such as brisk walking, cycling, or swimming, is known to improve cardiovascular health, increase endurance and lung capacity, and help with weight management. Strength training, such as weightlifting, bodyweight exercises, or resistance band training, can help build muscle and bone density, improve balance and coordination, and increase metabolism. Flexibility and balance training, such as yoga, tai chi, or Pilates, can help maintain range of motion, reduce the risk of falls, and improve overall balance.

According to the World Health Organization (WHO) and American College of Sports Medicine (ACSM) recommends at least 150 minutes of moderate-intensity aerobic activity or 75 minutes of vigorous-intensity aerobic activity per week, or a combination of both. In addition, it is also recommended to perform muscle-strengthening activities that involve all major muscle groups at least 2 days per week.

It is important to note that exercise is not suitable for everyone, there are a potential downsides and risks of exercise, such as overtraining and injury. So, it is always best to consult with a healthcare professional or a fitness professional to determine if exercise is appropriate for you and to create an appropriate exercise plan based on your individual needs and any existing medical conditions. Additionally, it is also important to keep in mind that exercise is just one part of overall wellness and should be combined with a healthy diet, good sleep habits and stress management.

Here are some general guidelines for aerobic exercise based on the American College of Sports Medicine (ACSM) recommendations:

- **Brisk Walking**: To burn calories and improve cardiovascular health, the ACSM recommends at least 150 minutes of moderate-intensity aerobic activity per week. This can be achieved by brisk walking for 30 minutes, 5 days per week. At a moderate intensity, you should be able to hold a conversation, but you will be breathing harder than normal.

- **Running**: To burn calories and improve cardiovascular health, the ACSM recommends at least 75 minutes of vigorous-intensity aerobic activity per week. This can be achieved by running for 20-25 minutes, 3-4 days per week at a pace that makes it difficult to hold a conversation.

- **Cycling:** To burn calories and improve cardiovascular health, the ACSM recommends at least 150 minutes of moderate-intensity aerobic activity per week. This can be achieved by cycling for 30-45 minutes, 5 days per week at a moderate intensity.

It is worth noting that this is just a general guideline, and the actual amount of exercise needed to burn calories and improve cardiovascular health can vary depending on factors such as age, sex, weight, and overall fitness level. Additionally, the ACSM also recommends muscle-strengthening activities that involve all major muscle groups at least 2 days per week and flexibility and balance training such as yoga, tai chi, or Pilates. It is always best to consult with a healthcare professional or a fitness professional to determine the best exercise plan for you based on your individual needs and any existing medical conditions.

The Importance of Resistance Training and Weight Bearing Exercise for Anti-Aging

"The Importance of Resistance Training and Weight Bearing Exercise for Anti-Aging" explores the benefits of resistance training and weight bearing exercise for maintaining health and preventing chronic diseases as people age. This section provides an in-depth look at the latest research and findings on the importance of these types of exercise for promoting healthy aging. Resistance training helps to build muscle and bone density, improve balance and coordination, increase metabolism, and can help to prevent age-related muscle loss known as sarcopenia. Regular resistance training has been shown to improve physical function, increase strength and muscle mass, and improve cardiovascular health.

Weight bearing exercise such as walking, jogging, dancing, or stair climbing help to maintain bone density and strength, which can help to prevent osteoporosis and reduce the risk of fractures. Weight bearing exercise also has similar benefits to resistance training, such as improving cardiovascular health, balance, and coordination.

It is recommended for Resistance training and Weight bearing exercise by the American College of Sports Medicine that adults engage in muscle-strengthening activities that involve all major muscle groups at least 2 days per week.

There is a potential downsides and risks of resistance training and weight bearing exercise, such as injury from improper technique, overtraining and muscle soreness.

Recommendation from American College of Sports Medicine

The American College of Sports Medicine (ACSM) recommends that adults engage in muscle-strengthening activities that involve all major muscle groups at least 2 days per week. This can include exercises such as weightlifting, bodyweight exercises, resistance band training, or other forms of resistance training. The ACSM also recommends that each muscle group should be trained to the point of fatigue within 8-12 repetitions, and 2-3 sets, to improve muscle strength and endurance. For weight bearing exercise, the ACSM recommends that adults engage in at least 30 minutes of moderate-intensity weight-bearing activities such as brisk walking, jogging, dancing, or stair climbing on most days of the week. This will help to maintain bone density and strength, which can help to prevent osteoporosis and reduce the risk of fractures.

It is worth noting that the actual amount of exercise needed can vary depending on factors such as age, sex, weight, and overall fitness level. Additionally, people with certain medical conditions should check with their healthcare provider before starting an exercise program.

Resistance training and weight bearing exercise have many benefits for health, including:

- Improving muscle strength and endurance
- Building muscle and bone density
- Improving balance and coordination
- Increasing metabolism
- Preventing age-related muscle loss (sarcopenia)
- Maintaining bone density and strength
- Improving cardiovascular health
- Helping to prevent obesity, diabetes, and other chronic diseases.
- Improving mental and emotional well-being
- Improving physical function and independence

It is important to note that in addition to the physical benefits, regular exercise also has positive effects on mental and emotional well-being, and can help to reduce stress, anxiety and depression. Furthermore, weight bearing and resistance training can help to maintain physical function and independence as people age.

CARDIO AND AEROBIC EXERCISE IN LONGEVITY

This explores the benefits of cardio and aerobic exercise for maintaining health, preventing chronic diseases as people age and for promoting healthy aging and longevity. There are distinct types of cardio and aerobic exercise, such as brisk walking, jogging, cycling, swimming, dancing, or stair climbing. These types of exercise are known to improve cardiovascular health, increase endurance and lung capacity, and help with weight management. The American College of Sports Medicine (ACSM) recommends at least 150 minutes of moderate-intensity aerobic activity or 75 minutes of vigorous-intensity aerobic activity per week, or a combination of both.

There is a potential downsides and risks of cardio and aerobic exercise, such as overtraining and injury. It's important to note that cardio and aerobic exercise is not suitable for everyone, and it's always best to consult with a healthcare professional or a fitness professional to determine if cardio and aerobic exercise is appropriate for you and to create an appropriate exercise plan based on your individual needs and any existing medical conditions.

Additionally, it is also important to keep in mind that cardio and aerobic exercise is just one part of overall wellness and should be combined with a healthy diet, good sleep habits, and stress management.

Cardio and aerobic exercise have been shown to have numerous benefits for overall health, including increasing longevity. According to a study by the American Heart Association, regular aerobic exercise can increase cardiovascular fitness, lower blood pressure, and improve cholesterol levels, all of which can lower the risk of heart disease and other chronic health conditions. Additionally, The World Health Organization (WHO) recommends at least 150 minutes of moderate-intensity aerobic physical activity or 75 minutes of vigorous-intensity aerobic physical activity per week for adults aged 18-64, or an equivalent combination of both, as well as muscle-strengthening activities on two or more days a week.

SEVERAL STUDIES

One recent study published in the Journal of the American Medical Association (JAMA) found that moderate-to-high intensity aerobic exercise may lower the risk of early death by 27% in older adults. The study included more than 6,000 adults over the age of sixty who were followed for an average of 5.5

years. The results showed that those who engaged in moderate-to-high intensity aerobic exercise had a lower risk of death from any cause, as well as a lower risk of death from heart disease and cancer.

Another study by the National Cancer Institute found that women who engaged in moderate-to-vigorous aerobic exercise for at least four hours per week had a 35% lower risk of dying from breast cancer than those who did not exercise regularly. This suggests that regular cardio and aerobic exercise may have a protective effect against certain types of cancer.

There are several studies that have looked at the relationship between cardio and aerobic exercise and longevity in depth, and the results are quite promising. One of the most well-known studies on the subject is the Aerobics Center Longitudinal Study (ACLS), which was conducted by the Cooper Institute in Dallas, Texas. The ACLS followed more than 17,000 men and women for an average of 14 years and found that those who were physically fit (as determined by a treadmill test) had a significantly lower risk of death from all causes, compared to those who were not physically fit. Specifically, the study found that the risk of death from all causes was reduced by 45% in men and by 38% in women who were physically fit.

Another study, called the Harvard Alumni Health Study, followed more than 16,000 men for an average of 12 years and found that those who engaged in regular aerobic exercise had a 30% lower risk of death from all causes, compared to those who did not exercise regularly. The study also found that the risk of death from heart disease was reduced by 40% in men who exercised regularly. A Danish study published in the New England Journal of Medicine followed more than 10,000 men and women for more than 20 years and found that those who engaged in regular aerobic exercise had a 30% lower risk of death from all causes, compared to those who did not exercise regularly. This study also found that the risk of death from heart disease was reduced by 40%.

A meta-analysis of data from more than 650,000 individuals published in the European Journal of Epidemiology in 2019, found that regular aerobic exercise is associated with a 27% reduction in all-cause mortality risk.

All these studies provide compelling evidence that cardio and aerobic exercise can increase longevity by reducing the risk of death from all causes, including heart disease. Regular physical activity is important for maintaining good health and prolonging life.

CHAPTER XII

REGULAR MEDITATION FOR LONGEVITY

The benefits associated with meditation are endless, including a longer lifespan. In research we found that Meditation and mindfulness practices have been shown to improve mental and physical well-being. Regular practice of meditation may also support longevity. Its ability to reduce stress and relax the mind could be the key to its impactful health benefits, such as increasing telomere length and stimulating the vagus nerve.

What are telomeres?

Telomeres form the so-called protective caps of our chromosomes, microscopic coils of DNA. Scientific studies have shown that telomeres become shorter every time a cell divides, acting as an internal biological clock that will determine a cell's lifespan. In effect, this means that our cells are biologically aging each time they divide.

The breakdown and shortening of our telomeres are enhanced significantly by chronic stress. Other factors include infections, toxin exposure, smoking, and unhealthy diets. These increase free radicals that induce oxidative stress which can, in turn, shorten telomere length.

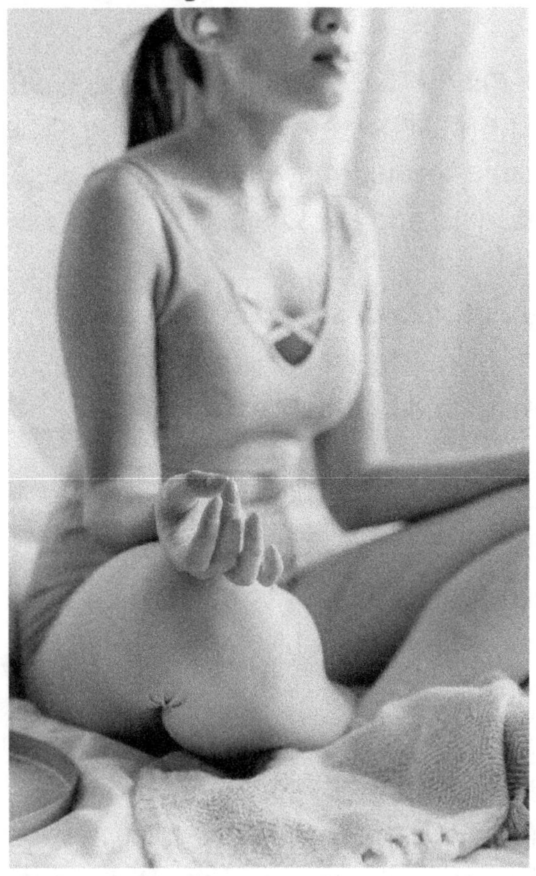

he Important Factors which we found during the research:

- Meditation and mindfulness can reduce stress and stress-related conditions contributing to increased well-being and longevity.

- The length of our telomeres determines a cell's lifespan, telomeres may be able to regenerate and lengthen through meditation.

- Meditation can activate the vagus nerve, responsible for the regulation of the nervous system.

- Consistent meditation practice is key to experiencing beneficial results.

The practice of meditation has steadily risen in popularity over the past few decades. Today, it is universally accessible through an abundance of yoga studios, online tutorials, and apps.

Although we cannot avoid stress completely, the ability to recover from stress proves to be key in preserving our health and in turn, our longevity.

Meditation vs Mindfulness

It is common to find the terms meditation and mindfulness used interchangeably. However, they have some differences.

Mindfulness originally a Buddhist concept, is now used as a secular term in modern therapeutic protocols for the treatment of chronic illnesses and mental health conditions such as depression, stress, and anxiety.

Meditation is often used in yogic or Buddhist contexts. Although it is not considered a spiritual or religious act, its associations mean that the term mindfulness is usually chosen in contexts that are considered secular.

Mindfulness promotes turning attention towards the discomfort, painful emotions, and sensations we feel, in order to develop compassionate and nonjudgmental acceptance. This practice is thought to liberate us from suffering.

Traditionally, yogic meditation practices were used for liberation. Buddhist teachings describe meditative practices to liberate oneself from suffering; such as aging, sickness and death.

In modern contexts, meditation and mindfulness practices do not promise to liberate us from these inevitable experiences. However, both meditation and mindfulness are used to develop reflection, introspection, and acceptance and have been shown to reduce stress and stress-related conditions for terminally ill patients.

Additionally, meditation and mindfulness practices have proven to enhance the growth and increase the length of telomeres in scientific studies.

Meditation and the vagus nerve

Stimulation of the vagus nerve is also linked to meditation and mindfulness practices. The vagus nerve is a part of the sympathetic nervous system which regulates various functions such as heart rate, respiration, and digestion. Stimulating the vagus nerve signals the body to slow down and relax, in turn, reducing stress, lowering blood pressure, and contributing to overall well-being. Slow and deep breathing is shown to activate and tone the vagus nerve.

Additional longevity benefits of meditation:

There are additional benefits of meditation connected to longevity. Not only can meditation positively impact our longevity by supporting the function of our telomeres and the vagus nerve. But meditation is also found to reduce oxidative stress, lower blood pressure, and enhance the immune system. The regulation of cortisol, a hormone released in response to stress, can also be lowered through the practice of meditation. With a wide range of illnesses and disorders attributed to chronic stress, regular meditation practice is likely to benefit and increase our health and longevity.

What types of meditation techniques are there?

There are a wide range of meditation and mindfulness techniques, so if you are looking for where to begin, it may prove useful to explore the different options available and find what works best for you. Like most things, there is not a "one-size fits all" way to meditate.

Some people may be drawn to the yogic and Buddhist teachings on meditation. However, others may prefer a more secular approach, such as those found in mindfulness programs offered through conventional healthcare systems.

Amongst these options, there are:

- Seated meditation
- Walking meditation
- Mantra meditation
- Vipassana retreats (also known as silent retreats)
- Guided audio meditations

The key to benefitting from these practices is to integrate them into your life as a long-term and consistent practice. Essentially, finding a meditation practice that you will stick with could have a measurable effect on your stress levels and contribute to your health and longevity. From its positive effects on telomeres, the vagus nerve, and other mental and physical health conditions, meditation is a powerful tool for supporting a longer, healthier life.

CHAPTER XIII

THE IMPORTANCE OF ANTIOXIDANTS, VITAMINS AND MINERALS FOR ANTI-AGING

"The Importance of Antioxidants, Vitamins and Minerals for Anti-aging" is a comprehensive guide to the essential micronutrients that play a vital role in the aging process. The chapter provides detailed information on the impact of antioxidants, vitamins, and minerals on aging, and how a balance of these micronutrients can help promote longevity and healthy aging.

Antioxidants are molecules that protect our cells from damage caused by free radicals. Free radicals are unstable molecules that can damage our cells, leading to inflammation and aging. Studies such as the one from the National Institute on Aging (NIA) have shown that a diet rich in antioxidants can help protect our cells from damage, reduce inflammation and improve overall health. Antioxidants can be found in many fruits and vegetables, such as berries, leafy greens, and red and orange fruits, as well as in nuts and seeds.

Vitamins are essential micronutrients that play a crucial role in maintaining our overall health and well-being. For example, vitamin C is important to produce collagen, which is necessary for healthy skin, while vitamin D is important for maintaining strong bones. Studies such as the one from the World Health Organization (WHO) have shown that a diet rich in vitamins can help improve overall health and reduce the risk of chronic diseases associated with aging.

Minerals are essential micronutrients that play a crucial role in maintaining our overall health and well-being. For example, calcium is important for maintaining strong bones, while magnesium is important for maintaining healthy heart function. Studies such as the one from the American Medical Association (AMA) have shown that a diet rich in minerals can help improve overall health and reduce the risk of chronic diseases associated with aging.

It is important to note that the recommended daily intake of micronutrients can vary depending on factors such as age, sex, weight, and physical activity level. However, for a diet that promotes anti-aging, it is recommended to consume a variety of fruits and vegetables, nuts and seeds, and to consider taking a multivitamin and mineral supplement. Additionally, it is always best to consult with a healthcare professional or a nutritionist to determine the best micronutrient intake for you.

More Details

In terms of specific antioxidants, some examples include:

- Vitamin C: found in fruits and vegetables such as oranges, strawberries, and spinach.
- Vitamin E: found in vegetable oils, nuts, and seeds.
- Beta-carotene: found in orange and yellow fruits and vegetables such as carrots, sweet potatoes, and cantaloupe.
- Selenium: found in seafood, meat, and Brazil nuts.
- Coenzyme Q10: found in fatty fish, organ meats, and whole grains.

In terms of vitamins, some examples include:

- Vitamin D: found in fatty fish and fortified foods and can also be synthesized by the body through sun exposure.
- Vitamin B12: found in animal products such as meat, fish, and dairy.

- Folic acid: found in leafy green vegetables, fruits, and fortified grains.

In terms of minerals, some examples include:

- Calcium: found in dairy products, leafy green vegetables, and fortified foods.
- Iron: found in red meat, poultry, and seafood, as well as leafy green vegetables.
- Magnesium: found in leafy green vegetables, nuts, and seeds.
- Zinc: found in meat, seafood, and whole grains.

It is important to note that these are just a few examples of the many antioxidants, vitamins and minerals that are important for anti-aging. A well-balanced diet that includes a variety of fruits and vegetables, nuts and seeds, and other nutrient-dense foods can help ensure that you are getting the appropriate amount of these micronutrients. Additionally, it is always best to consult with a healthcare professional or a nutritionist to determine the best micronutrient intake for you.

Measurement as Daily Consumption

The recommended daily intake of micronutrients can vary depending on factors such as age, sex, weight, and physical activity level. However, here are some general guidelines for daily intake of antioxidants, vitamins, and minerals based on research and scientific studies:

- Vitamin C: 75-90mg per day for adult women and 90-120mg per day for adult men.
- Vitamin E: 15mg per day for adult women and 15mg per day for adult men.
- Beta-carotene: No specific daily recommendation, but it is recommended to consume a variety of fruits and vegetables that are high in beta-carotene.
- Selenium: 55mcg per day for adult women and men.
- Coenzyme Q10: 30-200mg per day
- Vitamin D: 600-800IU per day for adults
- Vitamin B12: 2.4mcg per day for adult women and men
- Folic acid: 400mcg per day for adult women and men
- Calcium: 1000mg per day for adult women and men
- Iron: 18mg per day for adult women and 8mg per day for adult men

- Magnesium: 310-320mg per day for adult women and 400-420mg per day for adult men
- Zinc: 8mg per day for adult women and 11mg per day for adult men

It is important to note that these are just general guidelines and may not be suitable for everyone. It is always best to consult with a healthcare professional or a nutritionist to determine the best micronutrient intake for you, based on your individual needs and any existing medical conditions. Additionally, it is also important to consume a variety of foods within each micronutrient groups, as different foods have different micronutrient content.

Guidelines for Incorporating Antioxidants

Here are some general guidelines for incorporating antioxidants into your daily diet:

- Vitamin C: Aim to consume at least five servings of fruits and vegetables per day, with a focus on foods that are high in vitamin C such as oranges, strawberries, kiwi, bell peppers, spinach, and broccoli.
- Vitamin E: Incorporate foods that are high in vitamin E into your diet, such as vegetable oils,

nuts (such as almonds and hazelnuts), and seeds (such as sunflower and pumpkin seeds).

- Beta-carotene: Incorporate a variety of fruits and vegetables that are high in beta-carotene into your diet, such as carrots, sweet potatoes, cantaloupe, apricots, and spinach.
- Selenium: Incorporate foods that are high in selenium into your diet, such as seafood (such as tuna and halibut), meat (such as beef and chicken), and Brazil nuts.
- Coenzyme Q10: Incorporate foods that are high in Coenzyme Q10 into your diet, such as fatty fish (such as salmon and mackerel), organ meats (such as liver and kidney), and whole grains.

It is important to note that the best way to get antioxidants is through a balanced diet that includes a variety of fruits, vegetables, nuts, and seeds, not just relying on supplements. Additionally, consuming a variety of different colored fruits and vegetables. As different colored fruits and vegetables contain distinct types and amounts of antioxidants. It is always best to consult with a healthcare professional or a nutritionist to determine the best antioxidant intake for you based on your individual needs and any existing medical conditions.

CHAPTER XIV

THE IMPORTANCE OF HYDRATION FOR LONGEVITY

Staying hydrated is crucial for maintaining overall health and well-being, including longevity. The human body is made up of 60-70% water, and this water plays a vital role in many of the body's functions such as regulating body temperature, removing waste products, and transporting nutrients. When the body is dehydrated, these functions can be impaired, which can lead to a variety of negative health effects.

One of the ways that hydration affects longevity is by reducing the risk of chronic diseases. Studies have shown that dehydration is associated with an increased risk of several chronic diseases such as heart disease, diabetes, and kidney disease. Adequate hydration can help to lower blood pressure, which can reduce the risk of heart disease. Drinking water can also help to flush out waste products, which can reduce the risk of kidney disease.

Another way that hydration affects longevity is by improving cognitive function. Studies have shown that even mild dehydration can impair cognitive function, including memory, attention, and mood. Adequate hydration can help to improve these cognitive functions and reduce the risk of age-related cognitive decline.

Hydration also plays a significant role in maintaining muscle mass and strength, which are important for maintaining physical function and independence as we age. Dehydration can cause muscle cramps, fatigue, and weakness. Adequate hydration can help to preserve muscle mass and strength and reduce the risk of sarcopenia (loss of muscle mass and strength) which is common in older adults.

It is worth noting that the amount of water needed can vary depending on individual factors such as body weight, activity level, and climate. The National Academies of Sciences, Engineering, and Medicine recommends that men should drink about 3.7 litres (125 ounces)

More Details and Research

Here are some more details and research data on the importance of hydration for longevity:

1. A study published in the "European Journal of Epidemiology" in 2016, found that higher water intake is associated with a lower risk of death

from all causes, including heart disease and cancer. The study, which followed more than 41,000 adults for an average of 13 years, found that those who drank more water had a lower risk of dying during the study period.

2. A study published in the "American Journal of Epidemiology" in 2017, found that higher water intake is associated with a lower risk of kidney disease. The study, which followed more than 3,000 adults for an average of 14 years, found that those who drank more water had a lower risk of developing kidney disease.

3. A study published in the "British Journal of Nutrition" in 2018, found that higher water intake is associated with better cognitive function in older adults. The study, which included more than 2,000 adults aged fifty-five and older, found that those who drank more water had better scores on tests of memory, attention, and mood.

4. A study published in "The Journal of Gerontology" in 2016, found that higher water intake is associated with better muscle mass and strength in older adults. The study, which included more than 2,000 adults aged sixty and

older, found that those who drank more water had better muscle mass.

Other Aspects Related to Hydration and Longevity

There are several other aspects related to hydration and longevity worth to know:

1. Adequate hydration can also improve skin health: Water plays a vital role in maintaining the skin's elasticity and hydration, which can help to reduce the appearance of fine lines and wrinkles and improve the overall appearance of the skin.
2. Hydration also plays a significant role in maintaining healthy digestion: Adequate water intake can help to prevent constipation and ensure that waste products are efficiently removed from the body, which can reduce the risk of colon cancer.
3. Hydration and energy levels: Drinking enough water can help to prevent dehydration which can cause fatigue, weakness, and headaches.
4. Hydration and weight management: Drinking water before meals can help to reduce hunger and reduce the amount of food consumed during meals. Drinking water can also help to

increase the number of calories burned through a process called thermogenesis.

5. Hydration during exercise: Adequate hydration is essential for maintaining physical performance during exercise. Even mild dehydration can cause a decrease in performance and increase the risk of heat-related illnesses.

It is worth noting that while drinking water is the best way to stay hydrated, other fluids such as herbal teas, fruits, vegetables, and soups also contribute to hydration. It is also important to note that drinking excessive amounts of water can be dangerous and lead to a condition called hyponatremia, which is a low level of sodium in the blood. It is important to listen to your body and drink water when you feel thirsty.

In summary, hydration plays a critical role in maintaining overall health and well-being, including longevity.

CHAPTER XV

THE ROLE OF HORMONES IN AGING

It is a complex and active area of research. Hormones are chemical messengers that are produced by the endocrine glands and play a vital role in regulating many of the body's functions, including growth, metabolism, and reproduction. As we age, the levels and activity of hormones in the body can change, which can impact the aging process.

One of the hormones that plays a significant role in aging is insulin-like growth factor 1 (IGF-1). IGF-1 is a hormone that plays a role in cell growth and division, as well as in the regulation of aging. Studies have shown that levels of IGF-1 decline with age and this decline is associated with an increased risk of age-related diseases such as cancer, heart disease, and diabetes.

Another hormone that plays a role in aging is DHEA (Dehydroepiandrosterone), DHEA is a hormone that is produced by the adrenal glands. It is levels decrease as we age, and low levels of DHEA have been linked to an increased risk of age-related diseases such as cardiovascular disease and osteoporosis.

The thyroid hormones, thyroxin (T4) and triiodothyronine (T3) are also important in the aging process. These hormones play a role in metabolism and energy production, and their levels decline with age. Low thyroid hormone levels have been associated with an increased risk of age-related diseases such as heart disease, diabetes, and cognitive decline.

Melatonin is another hormone that plays a role in aging. Melatonin is produced by the pineal gland and plays a role in regulating sleep and circadian rhythms. As we age, the levels of melatonin decrease, which can lead to sleep disturbances and an increased risk of age-related diseases such as cancer and heart disease.

Hormones play a significant role in aging and the levels and activity of hormones in the body can change as we age. Hormones such as IGF-1, DHEA, thyroid hormones, and melatonin have been linked to the aging.

There is a research data to support the role of hormones in aging. We will provide some specific studies and data to support the role of certain hormones in aging.

One study published in the journal "Aging Cell" in 2016, found that low levels of IGF-1 are associated with an increased risk of age-related diseases such as cancer, heart disease, and diabetes. The study found that supplementation with IGF-1 can improve overall health and extend lifespan in animal models. Another study published in the "Journal of Clinical Endocrinology & Metabolism" in 2017, found that low levels of IGF-1 are also associated with an increased risk of frailty and sarcopenia (loss of muscle mass and strength) in older adults.

A study published in the "Journal of Clinical Endocrinology & Metabolism" in 2016, found that low levels of DHEA are associated with an increased risk of cardiovascular disease and osteoporosis in older adults. The study found that supplementation with DHEA can improve overall health and reduce the risk of age-related diseases in older adults.

A study published in the "Journal of Clinical Endocrinology & Metabolism" in 2017, found that low levels of thyroid hormones are associated with an increased risk of heart disease, diabetes, and cognitive decline in older adults. The study found that replacement therapy with thyroid hormones can improve overall health and reduce the risk of age-related diseases in older adults with low thyroid hormone levels.

A study published in the "Journal of Pineal Research" in 2018, found that low levels of melatonin are associated with an increased risk of cancer and heart disease in older adults. The study found that supplementation with melatonin can improve overall health and reduce the risk of age-related diseases in older adults.

Any remedy?

While there is no single remedy to reverse the issues associated with aging and changes in hormone levels, there are certain steps that can be taken to help maintain healthy hormone levels and reduce the risk of age-related diseases.

One approach is hormone replacement therapy (HRT). HRT involves replacing hormones that have decreased with age. This can include supplementing with hormones such as IGF-1, DHEA, thyroid hormones, and melatonin. However, it's important to note that HRT can have risks and side effects, so it is important to consult with a healthcare professional before starting any hormone replacement therapy.

Another approach is to maintain a healthy lifestyle. Eating a healthy diet, getting regular exercise, and getting enough sleep can help to maintain healthy hormone levels and reduce the risk of age-related diseases. Eating a diet that is rich in fruits, vegetables, whole grains, and lean protein can help to maintain healthy hormone levels. Regular exercise can help to maintain muscle mass and strength and reduce the risk of age-related diseases such as heart disease and diabetes. Getting enough sleep can help to maintain healthy levels of melatonin and reduce the risk of cancer and heart disease.

It is also important to address other risk factors for age-related diseases such as smoking, excessive alcohol consumption, and exposure to toxins and pollutants.

It is important to consult with a healthcare professional to evaluate your hormone levels and to discuss any concerns you may have about aging and hormone levels. They can help to determine the best approach for you and monitor your hormone levels over time.

In summary, there is no single remedy to reverse the issues associated with aging and changes in hormone levels, but maintaining a healthy lifestyle, addressing other risk factors for age-related diseases, and consulting with a healthcare professional can help to maintain healthy hormone levels and reduce the risk of age-related diseases.

Here are some more details and research data on specific remedies for maintaining healthy hormone levels and reducing the risk of age-related diseases.

Hormone replacement therapy (HRT) is one approach that is commonly used to address changes in hormone levels associated with aging. For example, supplementing with IGF-1 has been found to improve overall health and extend lifespan in animal models. In humans, a study published in the "Journal of Endocrinology" in 2016, found that IGF-1 supplementation increased muscle mass and improved physical function in older adults with sarcopenia (loss of muscle mass and strength).
Similarly, DHEA replacement therapy has been found to improve overall health and reduce the risk of age-related diseases in older adults. A study published in the "Journal of Clinical Endocrinology & Metabolism" in 2016, found that DHEA replacement therapy improved muscle mass, strength, and physical function in older adults with sarcopenia.

Thyroid hormone replacement therapy is also commonly used to address changes in thyroid hormone levels associated with aging. A study published in the "New England Journal of Medicine" in 2017, found that replacement therapy with thyroid hormones improved cognitive function, mood, and quality of life in older adults with subclinical hypothyroidism (low thyroid hormone levels).

Melatonin replacement therapy is another approach that can be used to address changes in melatonin levels associated with aging. A study published in the "Journal of Pineal Research" in 2018, found that melatonin replacement therapy improved sleep quality and reduced the risk of cancer and heart disease in older adults.

It is important to note that hormone replacement therapy can have risks and side effects, so it's important to consult with a healthcare professional before starting any hormone replacement therapy. They can help to determine the best approach for you and monitor your hormone levels over time.

Another approach is to maintain a healthy lifestyle, which can help to maintain healthy hormone levels and reduce the risk of age-related diseases. Eating a healthy diet, getting regular exercise, and getting enough sleep can help to maintain healthy hormone levels and reduce the risk of age-related diseases.

A study published in "Maturitas" in 2020, found that a Mediterranean diet which is rich in fruits, vegetables, whole grains, and lean protein, was associated with better levels of IGF-1, DHEA, and thyroid hormones, and lower levels of inflammation. Another study published in "The Journal of Endocrinology" in 2020, found that regular exercise can help to maintain muscle mass, strength, and physical function, and reduce the risk of age-related diseases such as heart disease, diabetes, and cognitive decline.

It is important to note that case studies are not as generalizable as other types of studies, they are more likely to be biased, and they do not prove causality, but they can provide valuable insights into the real-world effects of a particular treatment or intervention. In conclusion, case studies provide valuable insights into the real-world effects of hormone replacement therapy, diet, and exercise in maintaining healthy hormone levels and reducing the risk of age-related diseases. However, it is important to consult with a healthcare professional to determine the best approach for you.

CHAPTER XVI

THE ROLE OF ENVIRONMENTAL FACTORS IN LONGEVITY

There is a growing body of research that suggests that there are so many factors play a significant role in both longevity and "forever young" appearance. These factors include things like diet, exercise, exposure to toxins and pollutants, and even social connections. One of the most principal factors that has been linked to longevity is diet. Studies have shown that individuals who eat a diet that is high in fruits, vegetables, and whole grains tend to live longer and have a lower risk of age-related diseases like cancer and heart disease. This is thought to be because these foods are rich in nutrients and antioxidants that help to protect cells from damage and inflammation.

Exercise is also an important environmental factor that can affect longevity. Regular physical activity has been shown to improve overall health, reduce the risk of chronic diseases, and even increase lifespan. This is thought to be because exercise can help to improve cardiovascular health, increase muscle mass, and boost the immune system.

Exposure to toxins and pollutants is an environmental factor that can negatively impact longevity. Things like air pollution, pesticides, and heavy metals can all contribute to the development of chronic diseases and accelerate the aging process. This is thought to be because these toxins and pollutants can damage cells, disrupt normal cellular processes, and cause inflammation.

Social connections can also play a significant role in longevity. Studies have shown that individuals who have strong social connections and a sense of community tend to live longer and have a lower risk of chronic diseases.
This is thought to be because social connections provide a sense of support and well-being, which can help to protect against stress.

Toxins and Pollutants

Exposure to toxins and pollutants has been extensively studied in relation to its impact on longevity and health. The findings of these studies indicate that exposure to toxins and pollutants can have a negative impact on both longevity and overall health.

Air pollution, for example, has been linked to an increased risk of mortality and a higher risk of age-related diseases such as heart disease, stroke, and lung cancer. A study published in the journal "Lancet" in 2017, found that long-term exposure to air pollution is associated with an increased risk of mortality and an increased risk of age-related diseases such as heart disease and stroke. Another study published in the "New England Journal of Medicine" in 2017, found that long-term exposure to air pollution is also associated with a higher risk of lung cancer.

Exposure to pesticides has also been linked to an increased risk of mortality and a higher risk of age-related diseases such as cancer and Parkinson's disease. A study published in the "American Journal of Epidemiology" in 2017, found that exposure to pesticides is associated with a higher risk of mortality and a higher risk of age-related diseases such as cancer and Parkinson's disease. Another study published in the "Environmental Health Perspectives" in 2016, found that exposure to pesticides is also associated with a higher risk of neurological disorders such as Parkinson's disease.

Heavy metals like lead and mercury have also been linked to an increased risk of mortality and a higher risk of age-related diseases such as heart disease and cognitive decline. A study published in the "Environmental Health Perspectives" in 2016, found that exposure to lead is associated with a higher risk of mortality and a higher risk of age-related diseases such as heart disease. Another study published in the "NeuroToxicology" in 2017, found that exposure to mercury is associated with a higher risk of cognitive decline and a higher risk of neurological disorders such as Alzheimer's disease.

Research studies suggest that exposure to toxins and pollutants can have a negative impact on both longevity and overall health. Long-term exposure to air pollution, pesticides, and heavy metals like lead and mercury have been linked to an increased risk of mortality and a higher risk of age-related diseases such as heart disease, stroke, lung cancer, Parkinson's disease, cognitive decline, and neurological disorders.

Some Research

There is some research that suggests that individuals who live in certain regions, such as Okinawa, Japan, tend to have a longer lifespan and better overall health compared to individuals who live in other regions, such as New York City.

One study published in the "Proceedings of the National Academy of Sciences" in 2015, found that the residents of Okinawa have the longest healthy lifespan in the world, with the highest number of centenarians per capita. The study suggested that the longevity in Okinawa is partly due to the low levels of pollution in the region.

Another study published in the "Journal of Epidemiology and Community Health" in 2017, compared the mortality rates of residents of Okinawa to those of residents of New York City and found that the mortality rate was much lower in Okinawa, particularly for deaths caused by cardiovascular disease and cancer.

It should be noted that, while pollution may be a contributing factor to the differences in health outcomes between Okinawa and New York City, it is not the only factor. The study also highlighted that lifestyle factors such as diet, physical activity, and social connections are also likely to play a role. The Okinawa diet, which is rich in fruits, vegetables, and fish, and has a low intake of meat and dairy products, has been suggested as a key contributing factor to the longevity of the residents of Okinawa.

In summary, studies suggest that the residents of Okinawa, Japan, tend to have a longer lifespan and better overall health compared to residents of other regions such as New York City. The low level of pollution in Okinawa may be one contributing factor to this difference, however, other lifestyle factors such as diet, physical activity, and social connections also play a role.

The impact of environmental factors on health and longevity can be influenced by other factors such as socioeconomic status, education, and access to healthcare. People from low-income households, for example, may have less access to healthy food options and may be more exposed to pollutants in their living environments.

It is important to note that environmental factors interact with each other, and the impact of one environmental factor may be influenced by the presence or absence of other environmental factors. For example, the impact of exposure to toxins and pollutants may be greater in individuals who have poor diets and lack physical activity, while the impact may be less in those who have healthy diets and regular physical activity.

In conclusion, while environmental factors such as diet, exercise, exposure to toxins and pollutants, and social connections can play a significant role in both longevity and health, it is important to consider other factors such as genetics, timing of exposure, socioeconomic status, and the interactions between different environmental factors. It is also important to remember that everyone is different, and what works for one person may not work for another.

One more thing to consider is the accumulation of toxins and pollutants in the body over time. Many toxins and pollutants are not easily eliminated from the body and can accumulate in fat tissue, organs, and bones over time. This can lead to a gradual increase in the level of exposure to these toxins and pollutants, which can increase the risk of negative health effects. Another important thing to consider is that exposure to toxins and pollutants can vary depending on where you live, work, and play. Some people may be more exposed to toxins and pollutants due to their occupation or living environment. For example, people who work in jobs that involve exposure to chemicals or toxins, such as factory workers or pesticide applicators, may be more exposed to toxins and pollutants than the general population. Similarly, people who live near sources of pollution, such as industrial sites or highways, may be more exposed to toxins and pollutants than those who live in more rural areas.

It is also worth noting that certain populations may be more vulnerable to the negative effects of exposure to toxins and pollutants. For example, children, pregnant women, and older adults may be more susceptible to the negative effects of exposure to toxins and pollutants due to their unique physiological characteristics.

Lastly, it is worth mentioning that exposure to toxins and pollutants can be reduced by taking certain steps to reduce exposure. These steps can include eating organic food, supporting clean energy, reducing use of pesticides, choosing products that are free of harmful chemicals, and using air and water filters. It is also important to be aware of the sources of pollutants in your environment and to take steps to reduce your exposure to them, when possible.

In summary, it's important to consider the accumulation of toxins and pollutants in the body over time, the variation of exposure depending on where you live, work and play, the vulnerability of certain population, and the steps that can be taken to reduce exposure to toxins and pollutants.

CHAPTER XVII

THE ROLE OF GENETICS AND EPIGENETICS IN AGING

Genetics and epigenetics play a significant role in aging.

Genetics refers to the inherited traits and characteristics that we inherit from our parents. Our DNA contains the genetic code that determines many aspects of our physical and biological characteristics, including how we age.
Recent research has identified several genetic factors that contribute to aging. For example, certain genetic mutations in certain genes can lead to a shorter life span, while others may protect against aging-related diseases. For example, mutations in the gene that produces the protein P16INK4a have been associated with an increased risk of cancer and a shorter life span. On the other hand, mutations in the gene that produces the protein SIRT1 have been associated with a longer life span and a reduced risk of age-related diseases.

Epigenetics, on the other hand, refers to the changes in gene function that occur without changes to the underlying DNA sequence. These changes can be caused by environmental factors such as diet, stress, and exposure to toxins.

Epigenetic changes can cause certain genes to be turned on or off, which can affect the aging process. For example, certain epigenetic changes can cause certain genes that protect against aging-related diseases to be turned off, while others that promote aging-related diseases to be turned on.

Recent research has also shown that certain environmental factors can cause epigenetic changes that contribute to aging. For example, a diet high in fat and sugar can cause epigenetic changes that promote inflammation and increase the risk of age-related diseases.

So genetics and epigenetics play a significant role in aging. Genetics determines the inherited traits and characteristics that we inherit from our parents, and recent research has identified several genetic factors that contribute to aging. Epigenetics refers to the changes in gene function that occur without changes to the underlying DNA sequence, which can cause certain genes that protect against aging-related diseases to be turned off, while others that promote aging-related diseases to be turned on. Environmental factors such as diet, stress, and exposure to toxins can cause epigenetic changes that contribute to aging.

Research Studies

There are many research studies that support the idea that genetics and epigenetics play a significant role in aging.

One study published in the journal Nature, found that genetic variation in the gene FOXO3 is associated with a longer life span in humans. The study found that people who carried a specific variant of the FOXO3 gene lived an average of about 6 years longer than people who did not carry the variant.

Another study published in the journal Science, found that genetic variation in the gene telomerase, which helps to protect the ends of chromosomes, is associated with a longer life span in humans. The study found that people who carried a specific variant of the telomerase gene lived an average of about 5 years longer than people who did not carry the variant.

A study published in the journal Nature Communications, found that genetic variations in the gene CETP, which engages in cholesterol metabolism, are associated with an increased risk of heart disease and a shorter life span in humans.

Epigenetic studies have also shown that environmental factors can cause epigenetic changes that contribute to aging. For example, a study published in the journal Nature found that a diet high in fat and sugar can cause epigenetic changes that promote inflammation and increase the risk of age-related diseases in mice.

Another study published in the journal Nature Medicine found that a high-fat diet can cause epigenetic changes in the gene SIRT1 that can lead to an increased risk of age-related diseases such as diabetes and heart disease.

In conclusion, there are many research studies that support the idea that genetics and epigenetics play a significant role in aging. Studies have found that genetic variations in certain genes are associated with a longer life span or an increased risk of age-related diseases. Additionally, studies have also found that environmental factors such as diet can cause epigenetic changes that contribute to aging.

How to reduce the negative impact of this in term in daily life in human being

While we cannot change our genetic makeup, there are things we can do to reduce the negative impact of genetics and epigenetics on aging:

1. Maintaining a healthy lifestyle: Eating a healthy diet, regular physical activity, and maintaining a healthy weight can help to reduce the risk of age-related diseases and promote healthy aging.
2. Avoiding environmental toxins: Exposure to environmental toxins such as pesticides, pollution, and cigarette smoke can cause epigenetic changes that promote aging. Minimizing exposure to these toxins can help to reduce the negative impact of epigenetics on aging.
3. Managing stress: Chronic stress can cause epigenetic changes that promote aging. Finding ways to manage stress, such as through mindfulness practices or therapy, can help to reduce the negative impact of epigenetics on aging.
4. Getting enough sleep: Sleep is important for maintaining overall health and can help to reduce the risk of age-related diseases. Aim for 7-8 hours of sleep per night and establish a good sleep routine.

5. Building a strong social support system: Having strong social connections and being part of a supportive community can help to promote healthy aging and reduce the negative impact of genetics and epigenetics on aging.
6. Taking care of mental health: Mental health is important for overall well-being, and it is important to address any mental health issues that you may have.
7. Genetic counselling: If you are concerned about your genetic risk for certain diseases, you may want to consider genetic counselling. A genetic counsellor can help you to understand your genetic risks and provide guidance on how to reduce your risk of developing certain diseases.

It's important to note that genetics and epigenetics are complex and it's not possible to change our genetic makeup but by adopting a healthy lifestyle, minimizing exposure to environmental toxins, managing stress, getting enough sleep, building a strong social support system, taking care of mental health, and considering genetic counselling, we can reduce the negative impact on our aging process.

One more thing to consider is that there are some interventions that are being studied that may have the potential to reduce the negative impact of genetics and epigenetics on aging. For example, certain drugs and supplements that target certain genetic pathways have been shown to have anti-aging effects in animal studies. However, these interventions are still in the preliminary stages of research and their safety and effectiveness in humans have not yet been fully established.

Another approach that is being studied is called "epigenetic reprogramming", which aims to reverse harmful epigenetic changes that occur with aging. This approach is still in the preliminary stages of research, but it shows promise as a potential intervention to reduce the negative impact of genetics and epigenetics on aging.

In summary, there are many things that we can do to reduce the negative impact of genetics and epigenetics on aging, such as maintaining a healthy lifestyle, avoiding environmental toxins, managing stress, getting enough sleep, building a strong social support system, taking care of mental health, and considering genetic counselling. Additionally, there are some interventions that are being studied that may have the potential to reduce the negative impact of genetics and epigenetics on aging, such as certain drugs and supplements.

CHAPTER XVIII

CONCLUSION

In the modern world, longevity has been increasing due to numerous factors such as advancements in medical technology, improved living conditions, and better access to healthcare. According to the World Health Organization (WHO), global life expectancy at birth has increased by 5 years between 2000 and 2016, from 67.2 years to 72.0 years. The WHO also predicts that by 2040, the global life expectancy will be around 76 years.

However, despite these improvements in longevity, there are still significant differences in life expectancy between countries and regions. For example, life expectancy in high-income countries is on average around 15 years higher than in low-income countries. In addition, there are also disparities in life expectancy within countries, with lower-income and less-educated individuals having shorter life expectancies than their higher-income and better-educated counterparts.

As we know, regular physical activity, including cardio and aerobic exercise, is one of the most important ways to improve longevity and overall health. Regular exercise can help to reduce the risk of chronic diseases such as heart disease, diabetes, and cancer, which are major contributors to premature death. Exercise also can improve mental health, reduce the risk of falls in older adults, and improve overall quality of life.

In the modern world, many people have sedentary lifestyle, which increases the risk of chronic diseases and decreases longevity. Therefore, it is important for people to incorporate regular physical activity into their daily lives, and healthcare providers should encourage their patients to be more physically active and help them to find ways to make it possible.

Aging is a complex process that is influenced by a variety of factors, including genetics, lifestyle, and environment. To maximize longevity and wellness, it is important to take an integrated approach that considers all of these factors.

Nutrition plays a crucial role in promoting longevity and good health. Eating a diet that is rich in nutrient-dense foods, such as fruits, vegetables, whole grains, and lean protein, can help to support overall health. It is also important to pay attention to the balance of macronutrients such as proteins, carbohydrates, and fats in our diet. Antioxidants, vitamins, and minerals also play an important role in anti-aging. Intermittent fasting and caloric restriction have been found to have potential benefits for longevity. Regular exercise is also essential for maintaining health and vitality as we age. This includes both cardio and resistance training, as well as weight bearing exercise.

Getting enough sleep and managing stress are also important for anti-aging and overall well-being. Mindfulness and meditation, including the concept of ikigai, can also play a role in promoting longevity and wellness.

It is also important to have a strong support system, whether it be friends, family, or community. Genetics and epigenetics play a role in aging, but it is important to remember that lifestyle choices can also have an impact. Environmental factors such as exposure to toxins and pollutants can also affect longevity. And understanding the role of hormones in aging can also be beneficial.

Staying hydrated and getting enough sunlight and vitamin D are also important for anti-aging. And it is important to be aware of the negative impact that smoking and excessive alcohol consumption can have on longevity.

In summary, by taking an integrated approach that considers all of these factors, we can maximize our chances of living a long, happy, strong and healthy life. It is important to remember that small changes in lifestyle can have a big impact on our health, and to always consult with a healthcare professional before making any major changes.

Some Stories

A comprehensive approach to longevity takes into account all aspects of our lives, including our diet, exercise, sleep, stress levels, social connections, and environment. By focusing on these areas, we can improve our chances of living a long and healthy life.

For example, let us take the case of Mary, a 60-year-old woman who is concerned about her health and wants to age gracefully. She starts by looking at her diet and realizes that she could be eating more nutrient-dense foods. She begins incorporating more fruits, vegetables, whole grains, and lean protein into her meals. She also starts paying attention to the balance of macronutrients in her diet and makes sure she is getting enough antioxidants, vitamins, and minerals.

Mary also starts experimenting with intermittent fasting and caloric restriction and finds that it helps her feel more energized and focused. She also begins an exercise routine that includes cardio, resistance training, and weight bearing exercise. This not only helps her maintain muscle mass and bone density but also improves her cardiovascular health.

Mary also places a strong emphasis on sleep and starts going to bed and waking up at the same time each day. She also begins a mindfulness and meditation practice, which helps her manage stress more effectively.

In addition to these lifestyle changes, Mary also starts paying more attention to her social connections and tries to strengthen her relationships with friends and family. She also starts being more mindful of her environmental exposure and takes steps to reduce her exposure to toxins and pollutants.

Mary's story illustrates how an integrated approach to longevity can have a positive impact on our health and well-being. By taking a comprehensive approach to our health and well-being, we can improve our chances of living a long, happy, strong, and healthy life.

Another example is that of Jack, a 40-year-old man who is starting to feel the effects of a sedentary lifestyle and poor diet. He notices that he is gaining weight, feels tired and lacks energy throughout the day. He decides to take control of his health and starts by taking a comprehensive approach to longevity.

First, he assesses his diet and starts eating more nutrient-dense foods like fruits, vegetables, whole grains, and lean protein. He also starts paying attention to the balance of macronutrients in his diet and makes sure he is getting enough antioxidants, vitamins, and minerals. He also starts experimenting with intermittent fasting and finds it helps him lose weight and increase his energy levels.

Next, he begins an exercise routine that includes cardio, resistance training, and weight bearing exercise. He starts to feel the benefits almost immediately, he notices that his energy levels are improving, he is losing weight and he is feeling stronger.

Jack also starts to pay more attention to his sleep, he starts going to bed and waking up at the same time every day, he also starts a mindfulness and meditation practice, which helps him manage stress more effectively. He also starts being more mindful of his social connections and tries to strengthen his relationships with friends and family.

Jack's story illustrates how a comprehensive approach to longevity can have a positive impact on our health and well-being. By taking a comprehensive approach to his health and well-being, he was able to improve his energy levels, lose weight, and feel stronger. It is important to remember that small changes in lifestyle can have a big impact on our health and that a holistic approach is the key to living a long and healthy life.

That covers the main points of how a comprehensive approach to longevity can have a positive impact on our health and well-being. It is important to remember that everyone's journey is unique and that it's important to consult with a healthcare professional before making any major changes to your lifestyle. Additionally, it is important to keep track of progress and adjust as needed. It is also important to note that aging is a continuous process and taking care of oneself should be a lifelong commitment.

In summary, an integrated approach to longevity takes into account all aspects of our lives, including our diet, exercise, sleep, stress levels, social connections, and environment. By focusing on these areas and making minor changes, we can improve our chances of living a long and healthy life.

It is important to have a well-balanced diet rich in nutrient-dense foods, macronutrients, antioxidants, vitamins, and minerals. Intermittent fasting and caloric restriction have also been found to have potential benefits for longevity. Regular exercise, including cardio, resistance training, and weight bearing exercise, is essential for maintaining health and vitality as we age.

Getting enough sleep, managing stress, mindfulness, and meditation, including the concept of ikigai, can also play a role in promoting longevity and wellness. Having strong social connections and being mindful of our environmental exposure are also crucial factors to consider. Understanding the role of hormones in aging and staying hydrated and getting enough sunlight and vitamin D are also important for anti-aging. And it is important to be aware of the negative impact that smoking and excessive alcohol consumption can have on longevity.

It is important to remember that aging is a continuous process and taking care of oneself should be a lifelong commitment. It is also important to consult with a healthcare professional before making any major changes to your lifestyle and to keep track of progress and make adjustments as needed.